T0259613

New Developments in Management of Vascular Pathology of the Upper Extremity

Editors

STEVEN L. MORAN
KARIM BAKRI
JAMES P. HIGGINS

HAND CLINICS

www.hand.theclinics.com

Consulting Editor
KEVIN C. CHUNG

February 2015 • Volume 31 • Number 1

ELSEVIER

1600 John F. Kennedy Boulevard • Suite 1800 • Philadelphia, Pennsylvania, 19103-2899

http://www.theclinics.com

HAND CLINICS Volume 31, Number 1
February 2015 ISSN 0749-0712, ISBN-13: 978-0-323-35440-0

Editor: Jennifer Flynn-Briggs
Developmental editor: Stephanie Carter

© **2015 Elsevier Inc. All rights reserved.**

This periodical and the individual contributions contained in it are protected under copyright by Elsevier, and the following terms and conditions apply to their use:

Photocopying
Single photocopies of single articles may be made for personal use as allowed by national copyright laws. Permission of the Publisher and payment of a fee is required for all other photocopying, including multiple or systematic copying, copying for advertising or promotional purposes, resale, and all forms of document delivery. Special rates are available for educational institutions that wish to make photocopies for non-profit educational classroom use. For information on how to seek permission visit www.elsevier.com/permissions or call: (+44) 1865 843830 (UK)/(+1) 215 239 3804 (USA).

Derivative Works
Subscribers may reproduce tables of contents or prepare lists of articles including abstracts for internal circulation within their institutions. Permission of the Publisher is required for resale or distribution outside the institution. Permission of the Publisher is required for all other derivative works, including compilations and translations (please consult www.elsevier.com/permissions).

Electronic Storage or Usage
Permission of the Publisher is required to store or use electronically any material contained in this periodical, including any article or part of an article (please consult www.elsevier.com/permissions). Except as outlined above, no part of this publication may be reproduced, stored in a retrieval system or transmitted in any form or by any means, electronic, mechanical, photo-copying, recording or otherwise, without prior written permission of the Publisher.

Notice
No responsibility is assumed by the Publisher for any injury and/or damage to persons or property as a matter of products liability, negligence or otherwise, or from any use or operation of any methods, products, instructions or ideas contained in the material herein. Because of rapid advances in the medical sciences, in particular, independent verification of diagnoses and drug dosages should be made.

Although all advertising material is expected to conform to ethical (medical) standards, inclusion in this publication does not constitute a guarantee or endorsement of the quality or value of such product or of the claims made of it by its manufacturer.

Hand Clinics (ISSN 0749-0712) is published quarterly by Elsevier Inc., 360 Park Avenue South, New York, NY 10010-1710. Months of publication are February, May, August, and November. Business and Editorial Offices: 1600 John F. Kennedy Blvd., Ste. 1800, Philadelphia, PA 19103-2899. Customer Service Office: 3251 Riverport Lane, Maryland Heights, MO 63043. Periodicals postage paid at New York, NY and at additional mailing offices. Subscription price is $390.00 per year (domestic individuals), $606.00 per year (domestic institutions), $194.00 per year (domestic students/residents), $445.00 per year (Canadian individuals), $691.00 per year (Canadian institutions), $530.00 per year (international individuals), $691.00 per year (international institutions), and $256.00 per year (international and Canadian students/residents). Foreign air speed delivery is included in all *Clinics* subscription prices. All prices are subject to change without notice. **POSTMASTER:** Send address changes to *Hand Clinics*, Elsevier Health Sciences Division, Subscription Customer Service, 3251 Riverport Lane, Maryland Heights, MO 63043. Customer Service (orders, claims, online, change of address): Elsevier Health Sciences Division, Subscription Customer Service, 3251 Riverport Lane, Maryland Heights, MO 63043. Tel: 1-800-654-2452 (U.S. and Canada); 314-447-8871 (outside U.S. and Canada). Fax: 314-447-8029. E-mail: journalscustomerservice-usa@elsevier.com (for print support); journalsonlinesupport-usa@elsevier.com (for online support).

Reprints. For copies of 100 or more of articles in this publication, please contact the Commercial Reprints Department, Elsevier Inc., 360 Park Avenue South, New York, New York 10010-1710. Tel.: 212-633-3874; Fax: 212-633-3820; E-mail: reprints@elsevier.com.

Hand Clinics is covered in *MEDLINE/PubMed (Index Medicus), Current Contents/Clinical Medicine, EMBASE/Excerpta Medica,* and *ISI/BIOMED.*

Contributors

CONSULTING EDITOR

KEVIN C. CHUNG, MD, MS
Chief of Hand Surgery, University of Michigan
Health System; Charles B. G. de Nancrede
Professor of Surgery, Section of Plastic
Surgery, Department of Surgery; Professor of
Orthopaedic Surgery; Assistant Dean for
Faculty Affairs; Associate Director of Global
REACH, Ann Arbor, Michigan

EDITORS

STEVEN L. MORAN, MD
Professor and Chair of Plastic Surgery,
Professor of Orthopedic Surgery, Department
of Orthopedics and Division of Plastic Surgery,
Mayo Clinic, Rochester, Minnesota

KARIM BAKRI, MBBS
Assistant Professor of Plastic Surgery, Division
of Plastic Surgery, Mayo Clinic, Rochester,
Minnesota

JAMES P. HIGGINS, MD
Director, Curtis Hand Center,
Greater Chesapeake Hand Specialists,
Lutherville, Maryland

AUTHORS

KARIM BAKRI, MBBS
Assistant Professor of Plastic Surgery, Division
of Plastic Surgery, Mayo Clinic, Rochester,
Minnesota

HARVEY CHIM, MD
Associate Professor of Plastic Surgery,
Division of Plastic Surgery, University of Miami
Medical Center, Miami, Florida

RANDALL R. DE MARTINO, MD, MS
Division of Vascular and Endovascular Surgery,
Department of Surgery, Mayo Clinic,
Rochester, Minnesota

TRISTAN DE MOOIJ, MD
Research Fellow, Department of Orthopedic
Surgery, Mayo Clinic, Rochester, Minnesota

AUDRA A. DUNCAN, MD
Professor of Surgery, Division of Vascular
and Endovascular Surgery, Mayo Clinic,
Rochester, Minnesota

BEATRICE L. GRASU, MD
The Curtis National Hand Center, MedStar
Union Memorial Hospital, Baltimore,
Maryland

JAMES P. HIGGINS, MD
Director, Curtis Hand Center,
Greater Chesapeake Hand Specialists,
Lutherville, Maryland

HELEN G. HUI-CHOU, MD
The Curtis National Hand Center, MedStar
Union Memorial Hospital, Baltimore,
Maryland

CHRISTOPHER M. JONES, MD
The Curtis National Hand Center, MedStar Union Memorial Hospital, Baltimore, Maryland

SANJEEV KAKAR, MD, MRCS, MBA
Associate Professor of Orthopedic Surgery, Division of Hand Surgery, Mayo Clinic, Rochester, Minnesota

RYAN D. KATZ, MD
Curtis National Hand Center, MedStar Union Memorial Hospital, Baltimore, Maryland

DEREK L. MASDEN, MD
Clinical Assistant Professor, Department of Plastic Surgery, Georgetown University Hospital, Division of Plastic Surgery, Hand Surgery, Washington Hospital Center, Washington, DC

MICHAEL A. McCLINTON, MD
The Curtis National Hand Center, MedStar Union Memorial Hospital, Baltimore, Maryland

WYNDELL H. MERRITT, MD, FACS
Clinical Professor of Surgery, Division of Plastic and Reconstructive Surgery, Virginia Commonwealth University, Richmond, Virginia; Clinical Professor of Surgery, Department of Plastic and Maxillofacial Surgery, University of Virginia, Charlottesville, Virginia

BRETT MICHELOTTI, MD
Plastic Surgery Resident, Division of Plastic Surgery, University of Pennsylvania Hershey Medical Center, Hershey, Pennsylvania

STEVEN L. MORAN, MD
Professor and Chair of Plastic Surgery, Professor of Orthopedic Surgery, Department of Orthopedics and Division of Plastic Surgery, Mayo Clinic, Rochester, Minnesota

MICHAEL S. MURPHY, MD
The Curtis National Hand Center, MedStar Union Memorial Hospital, Baltimore, Maryland

MICHAEL W. NEUMEISTER, MD, FRCSC, FACS
Professor, Chair, Institute for Plastic Surgery, Southern Illinois University School of Medicine, Springfield, Illinois

WILLIAM C. PEDERSON, MD, FACS
Fellowship Director, The Hand Center of San Antonio, Adjunct Professor of Surgery, University of Texas Health Science Center at San Antonio, San Antonio, Texas

MARCO RIZZO, MD
Professor of Orthopedics, Department of Orthopedics and Division of Plastic Surgery, Mayo Clinic, Rochester, Minnesota

JOHN SHUCK, MD
Plastic Surgery Resident, Department of Plastic Surgery, Georgetown University Hospital, Washington, DC

VICTOR W. WONG, MD
Curtis National Hand Center, MedStar Union Memorial Hospital, Baltimore, Maryland

Contents

 Video of the Allen test used to assess for ulnar versus radial dominance accompanies this article

Vascular pathology of the upper extremity requires consideration of constitutional, anatomic, and functional factors. The medical history and physical examination are essential. The Allen test can be performed alongside a handheld Doppler for arterial mapping. Useful studies include digital–brachial index measurements, digital plethysmography, laser Doppler, and color ultrasounds. Three-phase bone scintigraphy still plays a role in the evaluation of vascularity after of frostbite injury. Angiogram remains the gold standard radiographic instrument to evaluate vascular pathology of the upper extremity, but computed tomography and magnetic resonance scans have an increasing role in diagnosis of vascular pathology.

Distal arm and hand ischemia from vessel thrombosis or embolism remains a difficult clinical challenge. The causes of ischemia are variable and include connective tissue disease, embolism, atherosclerosis, and iatrogenic etiology. Although reports are limited, treatment with catheter-directed thrombolysis has favorable results in cases of acute thrombosis, with most patients (80%) demonstrating improvement. Digital amputation rates are less than 10% and the hand is often salvaged. Bleeding and access-site complications remain prevalent in patients undergoing intra-arterial thrombolysis. This review discusses etiology, treatment approaches, outcomes, and complications when thrombolytic therapy is used for distal arm and hand ischemia.

Raynaud phenomenon may be a primary disorder or associated with a variety of other autoimmune processes. Raynaud phenomenon produces digital vasospasm, which can lead to ischemia and ulceration. The treatment of Raynaud phenomenon has been difficult because multiple medical treatments have not provided uniform resolution of symptoms. Many patients have turned to surgery and sympathectomies for the treatment of unrelenting vasospasm. Botulinum toxin has been shown to be an effective alternative to surgery, with a single treatment being capable of resolving pain and healing ulcer. This article reviews the use of botulinum toxin for the treatment of Raynaud phenomenon.

Repetitive, high-stress, or high-impact arm motions can cause upper extremity arterial injuries. The increased functional range of the upper extremity causes increased stresses on the vascular structures. Muscle hypertrophy and fatigue-induced joint translation may incite impingement on critical neurovasculature and can cause vascular damage. A thorough evaluation is essential to establish the diagnosis in a timely fashion as presentation mimics more common musculoskeletal injuries. Conservative treatment includes equipment modification, motion analysis and adjustment, as well as equipment enhancement to limit exposure to blunt trauma or impingement. Surgical options include ligation, primary end-to-end anastomosis for small defects, and grafting.

Hypothenar hammer syndrome is a rare vascular condition resulting from injury to the ulnar artery at the level of Guyon canal. The ulnar artery at the wrist is the most common site of arterial aneurysms of the upper extremity and is particularly prone to injury. Signs and symptoms include a palpable mass, distal digital embolization to long, ring, or small fingers, pain, cyanosis, pallor, coolness, and recurrent episodes of vasospasm. Modalities for diagnosis, evaluation, and surgical planning include duplex study, contrast arteriography, and computerized tomographic angiography (CTA). Management includes medical, nonoperative, or operative treatments. Appropriate treatment options are reviewed.

Hand ischemia caused by vasculitis is a secondary finding in many autoimmune processes. Many of these autoimmune diseases are managed primarily with medications that can prevent the development of occlusive disease, tissue ischemia, and tissue loss. Unfortunately several disease conditions can be recalcitrant to medical management and can result in ischemic changes within the hand, which may require operative intervention. This article briefly reviews the major connective tissue disorders associated with vasculitis and vaso-occlusive disease of the hand, including scleroderma, lupus, and Buerger disease, and their surgical treatment.

Direct arterial bypass remains the best option in patients with terminal ischemia of the hand, if there is an adequate distal target vessel. In situ bypass is the procedure of choice in patients who are candidates for arterial bypass. Venous arterialization offers an option in patients in whom there is not adequate arterial runoff in the hand. Venous arterialization should be avoided in patients with significant wounds and/or active infection. In selected patients, microvascular omental transfer can offer an option for revascularization of the ischemic hand.

Vascular grafts, as either interpositional conduits or bypass grafts, can be used for revascularization procedures in the upper extremity. Vein grafts are more readily available and can be easier to harvest. Arterial grafts may provide superior patency

HAND CLINICS

RELATED INTEREST

Anesthesiology Clinics, September 2014 (Vol. 32, Issue 3)
Vascular Anesthesia
Charles C. Hill, *Editor*

DOWNLOAD
Free App!

Review Articles
THE CLINICS

NOW AVAILABLE FOR YOUR iPhone and iPad

Preface

New Developments in Management of Vascular Pathology of the Upper Extremity

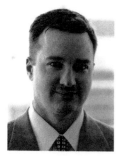
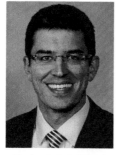
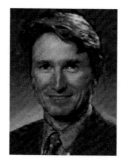

Steven L. Moran, MD   Karim Bakri, MBBS   James P. Higgins, MD

Editors

The management of vasospastic and vaso-occlusive disease of the upper extremity has been a challenging problem for the upper extremity surgeon for decades. A surprising 10% to 20% of premenopausal women suffer from cold sensitivity related to vasospasm.[1] In addition, the rising number of transradial endovascular procedures may soon increase the number of patients we see with acute and chronic hand ischemia related to radial artery trauma.

This issue of the *Hand Clinics* examines the diagnosis of occlusive and vasospastic disease in the manual laborer, athlete, and patient with connective tissue disease. We review the time-honored techniques of sympathectomy and arterial reconstruction in the management of these conditions as well as explore the use of newer treatment options, such as botulinum toxin for the management of Raynaud disease and catheter-directed thrombolytics for distal hand ischemia. In addition, we provide the most up-to-date review on vascular injury related to arterial lines and transradial catheterization. Our hope is to provide the reader with an up-to-date review of the evidence as well as the surgical pearls of world authorities on the management of vaso-occlusive disease.

The editors would like to thank all the contributing authors for their excellent articles. In addition, we would also like to offer a special thanks to Stephanie Carter for her tireless work in bringing this edition to fruition and to Dr Chung for allowing us to produce this issue of *Hand Clinics*.

Steven L. Moran, MD
Division of Hand Surgery
200 First Street, Mayo Clinic
Rochester, MN 55905, USA

Karim Bakri, MBBS
Division of Hand Surgery
200 First Street, Mayo Clinic
Rochester, MN 55905, USA

http://dx.doi.org/10.1016/j.hcl.2014.09.012
0749-0712/15/$ – see front matter © 2015 Elsevier Inc. All rights reserved.

hand.theclinics.com

James P. Higgins, MD
Greater Chesapeake Hand Specialists
1400 Front Avenue, Suite 100
Lutherville, MD 21093, USA

E-mail addresses:
Moran.steven@mayo.edu (S.L. Moran)
Bakri.karim@mayo.edu (K. Bakri)
jameshiggins10@hotmail.com (J.P. Higgins)

REFERENCE

1. Koman LA, Li Z, Smith BP. Vascular disorders: rational and basic science. In: Weiss AP, Goldfarb CA, Hentz VR, et al, editors. Textbook of hand and upper extremity surgery. Chicago: American Society of Surgery of the Hand; 2013. p. 1419.

Use of Diagnostic Modalities for Assessing Upper Extremity Vascular Pathology

Beatrice L. Grasu, MD, Christopher M. Jones, MD,
Michael S. Murphy, MD*

KEYWORDS

- Allen test • Digital–brachial index • Laser Doppler fluxometry • Color ultrasound
- Photoplethysmography • Cold stress testing • Angiography

KEY POINTS

- A diagnosis of vascular insufficiency begins with the history and physical examination, including systemic vascular diseases, digit and nail inspection, and the Allen test.
- The handheld Doppler and ultrasound are useful instruments to audibly and visually evaluate normal or obstructed vessels throughout the upper extremity.
- The vascular laboratory includes several crucial tests to evaluate vascular insufficiency including Doppler fluxometry, plethysmography, cold stress testing, and nail fold capillaroscopy.
- Angiography is the gold standard, but the evolution of computed tomography and magnetic resonance imaging have improved visualization of upper limb vessels in a noninvasive manner.

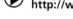 Video of the Allen test used to assess for ulnar versus radial dominance accompanies this article at http://www.hand.theclinics.com/

INTRODUCTION

Vascular pathology in the upper extremity includes a wide spectrum of pathology. Evaluation of vascular pathology of the upper extremity requires consideration of constitutional, anatomic, and functional factors. Beginning with a thorough history and physical examination and continuing with objective assessments such as laboratory testing and specialized studies in the vascular and radiology suites, an accurate diagnosis may be obtained. These specialized tests evaluating upper extremity blood vessels also assist in appropriate treatment recommendations.

Vascular disorders are much more common in the lower limb than the upper limb; however, upper extremity vascular disorders may be similarly debilitating. Vascular pathology may present as part of a systemic disorder affecting both extremities or as an isolated unilateral injury. Symptoms of cold sensitivity, signs of ulceration, skin changes such as hair loss, numbness, pain, and gangrene indicate inadequate nutritional flow to sustain the metabolic needs of distal soft tissues.[1]

The causes may involve physical obstruction or structural abnormalities, vasospastic disease, or a combination of both, termed vaso-occlusive disease. The primary goal of treatment is to restore

The authors have nothing to disclose.
The Curtis National Hand Center, MedStar Union Memorial Hospital, 3333 North Calvert Street, #200 JPB, Baltimore, MD 21218, USA
* Corresponding author.
E-mail address: mmurphy@chesapeakehand.com

0749-0712/15/$ – see front matter © 2015 Elsevier Inc. All rights reserved.

hand.theclinics.com

pulsatile blood flow to nutritional capillary beds. Diagnostic tools to determine structural or functional abnormalities within blood vessels are useful to decide on appropriate management.[1]

ANATOMY

The vascularity of the upper extremity is intricate. The arterial supply is derived from the subclavian artery, which originates from the brachiocephalic (innominate) artery on the right and directly from the aortic arch on the left. The subclavian artery gives off several branches to the head and neck before it becomes the axillary artery at the level of the first rib. After supplying branches to both the shoulder and scapula, the axillary artery becomes the brachial artery just below the axilla. The brachial artery travels medially down the arm and elbow to give off a deep branch and collateral vessels that provide an arterial anastomosis to the elbow. It then terminates just distal to the elbow in its bifurcation to the radial and ulnar arteries, which course along their respective sides of the forearm. The ulnar and radial arteries give off recurrent arteries to also provide collateral circulation around the elbow. The ulnar artery also gives off an interosseous branch that trifucates into posterior, recurrent, and anterior branches. Further distally, the ulnar artery becomes the superficial palmar arch, and the radial artery becomes the deep palmer arch. Both arches of the hand give off arterial branches to supply the thumb and fingers.[2]

The venous system of the upper extremity includes a superficial and deep network. Superficially, the cephalic vein is located more lateral in the upper arm, whereas the basilic vein is located more medially. These 2 veins typically join just distal to the elbow at the median antecubital vein. The deep system includes the radial and ulnar veins in the forearm, which unite caudal to the elbow to form the brachial veins. The brachial veins join the basilic vein, typically at the level of the teres major muscle, and continue as the axillary vein. The axillary vein passes through the axilla and crosses the first rib before becoming the lateral portion of the subclavian vein. The medial portion of the subclavian vein includes the external and internal jugular vein, which all flow into the brachiocephalic vein.

HISTORY AND PHYSICAL EXAMINATION FINDINGS

Determining abnormal vascular pathology begins with a complete history and physical examination. Patients may not report any symptoms from mild vascular disease; however, they may describe pain from repetitive use of their upper extremities causing intermittent claudication. As the disease progresses, pain and skin, nail, and hair changes may occur. Inquiries regarding past medical history, cardiac history, smoking use, and similar symptoms in the contralateral extremity or lower extremities are crucial.

The symptomatic extremity should be compared with the contralateral limb. There are many physical tests to evaluate vascular insufficiency in the upper extremity. Routine palpation of the radial, ulnar, and brachial pulses suggests intact arterial flow. Inspection of the skin for color or pallor, ulcerations, hair loss, or fingernail changes may uncover hallmark signs of embolic or other signs of chronic ischemia (**Fig. 1**).

The Allen test was first described in 1929 to diagnose occlusive disease of ulnar circulation in thromboangiitis obliterans.[1] It provides a means of assessment of the contribution of the ulnar artery and radial artery to the blood flow to the hand.

Allen Test

The test should be performed as follows (**Fig. 2**, Video 1)

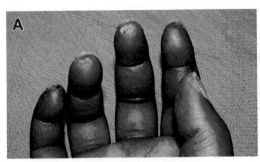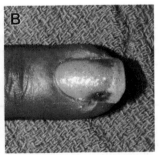

Fig. 1. Ischemic ulcerations at the tips of second through fifth digits prior to revascularization (*A*). Nail changes also known as splinter hemorrhages indicating digital vessel emboli and capillary ischemia (*B*). (*Courtesy of R.D. Katz, MD, Baltimore, MD.*)

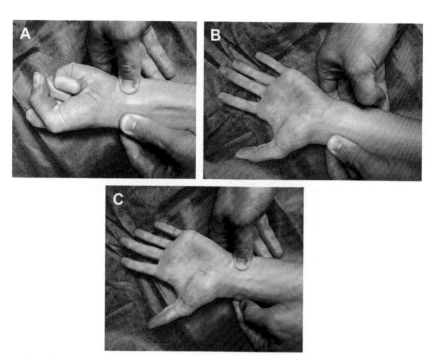

Fig. 2. Perform the Allen test to assess for ulnar versus radial dominance by compressing both the ulnar and radial arteries until the hand becomes pale (*A*). Then release pressure on the ulnar artery while maintaining compression on the radial artery (*B*). Evaluate for capillary perfusion and then repeat the test by reversing the compressed vessel (*C*).

- Elevate the hand and ask the patient to make a fist for 30 second to 1 minute.
- Apply pressure to both the radial and ulnar arteries to occlude them.
- With hand still elevated, ask the patient to open the fist; observe hand pallor.
- Release pressure off one of the arteries, but maintain pressure on the other.
- Study how long it takes for the color to return to the hand.
- Repeat the examination but reverse which artery remains occluded.

In 1981, Gelberman presented a technique for timing the return of blood flow to the palm to a quantitative element to arterial occlusion identification.[3] Evaluation of 800 hands showed the average fill time for the radial artery was 2.4 plus or minus 1.2 seconds and 2.3 plus or minus 1.0 seconds for the ulnar artery. If hand color returned in less than 6 seconds, the examination was considered within normal limits.[1] Interestingly, unlike ulnar artery aneurysms, radial artery aneurysms do not generally cause arterial occlusion, and so the Allen test might demonstrate a normal examination or flow through the radial artery even though pathology exists.

The Allen test can also be performed for each finger to assess digital artery patency (**Fig. 3**).

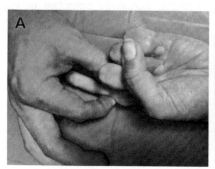
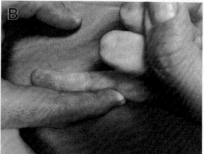

Fig. 3. (*A*) The Allen test can also be performed in the hand to assess radial and ulnar digital artery circulation by compressing both the radial and ulnar digital arteries. (*B*) Then release pressure off the ulnar digital artery to evaluate digital flow through the index finger.

The digital arteries are occluded at the base of the digit, and the hand is elevated. The finger is flexed several times to cause blanching, and then the hand is lowered. If the finger remains blanched after lowering the hand and releasing compression of 1 digital artery, then the released digital artery is considered compromised.[1]

In conjunction with the Allen test, the handheld Doppler is a useful tool to evaluate blood flow or velocity through the radial and ulnar arteries at the wrist and the digital arteries. The Doppler also allows mapping of the arterial network. There are several types of Doppler transducers to match specific requirements for physiologic application such as suction-on Doppler flow probes or suture-down transducers. Most commonly seen for evaluation of the upper extremity is the extra-vascular Doppler flow transducer. This transducer consists of a stainless steel tube with a 1 mm diameter piezoelectric crystal mounted at a 45° angle inside. For this reason, the probe should be angled at a 45° to the vascular bed while using conductive gel and avoiding excessive compression (**Fig. 4**). The reflected sound waves result from the movement of blood cells and vary with blood flow velocity. This velocity is visualized in a triphasic flow pattern if it is normal, whereas areas of occlusion or compression also have characteristic flow patterns (**Fig. 5**). There is no correlation between the arterial Doppler signal and systolic blood pressure or actual blood volume.[1] The Allen test may be performed while using the handheld Doppler to assess the arterial flow in the digits (**Fig. 6**).

Another useful physical examination test is the Adson maneuver: arm abduction and extension while rotating the patient's head to the ipsilateral elevated arm and extending the neck after deep

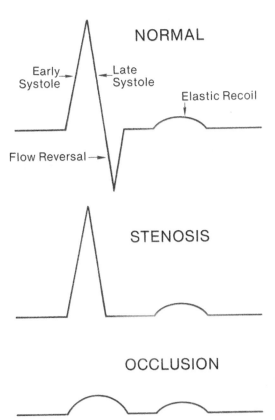

Fig. 5. Normal arterial waveform patterns of the Doppler signal have a triphasic pattern (*top*), while obstructed (*middle*) and stenotic (*bottom*) vessels have these characteristic patterns. Normal triphasic arterial wave form patterns are schematically depicted. The changes that occur with stenosis or occlusion are similarly depicted. (*From* Koman LA. Diagnostic study of vascular lesions. Hand Clin 1985;1(2):221; with permission.)

inspiration. The examiner palpates the radial pulse before and during the maneuver and if it decreases or is completely absent, the maneuver is positive for diagnosis of thoracic outlet obstruction. Patients frequently complain of vague, diffuse arm pain, or fatigue with activity, especially overhead exercises.

VASCULAR LABORATORY

More advanced vascular studies such as digital–brachial index, laser Doppler, ultrasound, digital plethysmography, digital pulse–volume recording (PVR), cold stress testing, and nail fold capillaroscopy can provide further clinical benefit.

Similar to ankle–brachial index, the digital–brachial index (DBI) is a ratio of the systolic pressure of the digit to the systolic brachial pressure. A miniature blood pressure cuff is placed on the

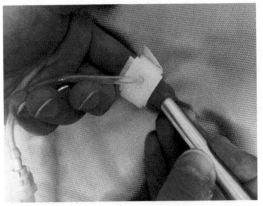

Fig. 4. Using a conductive gel, angle the Doppler probe about 45° to the vessel being studied.

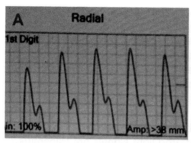
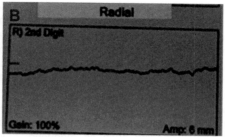

Fig. 6. Normal triphasic Doppler signal of the first digit while performing the Allen test and obstructing the radial artery (*A*). Evaluation of the second digit during Allen testing revealed an obstruction in the ulnar digital artery with this Doppler signal (*B*).

respective digit, and the systolic value is obtained (**Fig. 7**). Abnormally large pressure gradients between the two suggest structural, obstructive disease such as stenosis, thrombosis, or embolus. A ratio less than 0.7 is indicative of significant vascular disease, and treatment is encouraged.[1] A DBI of 0.5 suggests imminent digital gangrene. The examiner should be cautious of a normal or elevated index in a diabetic patient, because his or her vessels may be calcified or stiffer, falsely elevating absolute pressure assessments.

Laser Doppler fluxometry and perfusion imaging are other noninvasive tools available to evaluate vascular flow of the upper extremity. Laser Dopplers use laser lights to measure the flux (velocity × number of blood cells) or real-time cutaneous perfusion. Flow measurements reflect movement of capillary cells and blood flow in the peripheral thermoregulatory bed.[1] The laser Doppler perfusion imaging technique is a quantitative measurement of surface skin blood flow. A color-coded image of the tissue perfusion distribution is reproduced on a computer screen, which provides mean perfusion values.[1] Additional noninvasive evaluation with a color Duplex ultrasound can provide the examiner with real-time structural and functional vascular anomalies.

Ultrasound is the initial imaging modality to evaluate the upper extremity venous system. It can differentiate between deep and superficial veins; only deep veins have arteries running with them in the upper limb, and it is the deep venous system that is clinically important in cases of obstruction or thrombosis. The overlying clavicle and first rib make upper extremity ultrasound more technically challenging than the lower extremity. By adjusting the angle of the probe, such as an inferiorly angled supraclavicular approach, evaluation of the brachiocephalic vein and medial portion of the subclavian vein is possible. Valsalva maneuver or brisk inspiratory stiff results in normal venous collapse or narrowing and may assist in determining significant stenosis or obstruction of the deep, central venous system.[4] Color images may

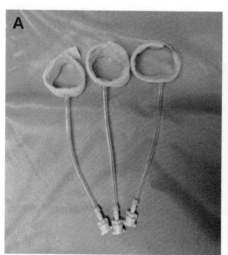
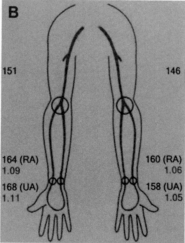

Fig. 7. Blood pressure cuffs to obtain systolic digital blood pressure (*A*). Useful in calculating DBI (*B*).

be acquired to appreciate real-time venous or arterial blood flow, and a corresponding Doppler signal can be obtained (**Fig. 8**). Ultrasound is indicated for assessment of dialysis access and intravenous access, venous mapping before harvest for arterial bypass, and determination or follow-up of venous thrombosis, aneurysm, or hematoma.[4,5] If sonographic findings are equivocal or nondiagnostic, especially in studies of the central deep veins, further imaging such as magnetic resonance venography may be useful.[5]

Plethysmography is the study of changes in volume of an organ from the fluctuations in blood or air it contains. Digital plethysmography, also known as the study of changes in digital blood volume, is assessed using air-filled cuffs connected to pressure transducers and photoplethysmographs (PPGs). This pulse–volume recording (PVR) is a functional test, meaning that it evaluates all of the blood flow to the examined extremity, not just a specific blood vessel. The surface area under the PVR waveform is entered into a spreadsheet and compared with and without arterial compression to calculate the pulse–volume ratio. A pulse–volume ratio close to zero indicates that this compressed artery is required for pulsatile flow to the digit, whereas a ratio of 1 or greater suggests that this artery is not required for digital blood flow.[6] Wilgis and colleagues studied the ulnar and radial arteries and their contributions to digital blood flow in patients undergoing coronary bypass grafting or radial forearm free flap. The results suggested that loss of radial flow with wrist compression causes more acute changes in pulsatile flow to the thumb, index, and small fingers than ulnar artery compression.

A transmitter–receiver unit usually less than 1 cm^2 is placed on the pulp of the tested digit to obtain PVRs. Using a light-emitting diode (LED), infrared light signals are transmitted and received from moving erythrocytes (**Fig. 9**).[7] Accordingly, it varies with changes in digital artery blood content and lumen dimension.[1,7] Similar to Doppler readings, the tracing of a normal artery should produce a triphasic wave pattern, whereas stenotic and occluded vessels will produce classic, pathognomonic waveform patterns (**Fig. 10**). Pre- and postoperative plethysmographs may be obtained to evaluate effectiveness of interventions, such as digital periarterial sympathectomy for scleroderma or severe Raynaud disease.

Digital temperature evaluation is a crude method to assess vascular flow. Cutaneous surface temperature of the digit is directly proportional to blood flow and normally ranges between 20°C and 30°C.[1] Temperature fluctuation should be taken into consideration because environmental conditions can affect isolated measurements. Isolated cold stress testing studies the ability of a vascular bed to respond to and

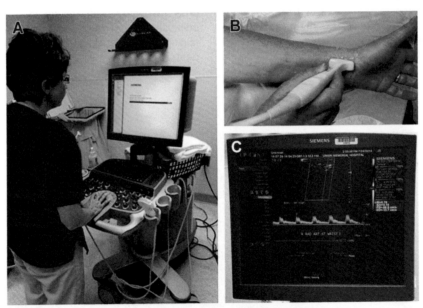

Fig. 8. Ultrasound is often the first noninvasive vascular study to evaluate pathology and is typically performed in the vascular suite by a trained technician (*A*). To obtain an image, use conductive gel and place the probe at about a 45° angle (*B*). Color ultrasound images may be acquired to appreciate real-time venous or arterial blood flow, and a corresponding Doppler signal can be obtained (*C*).

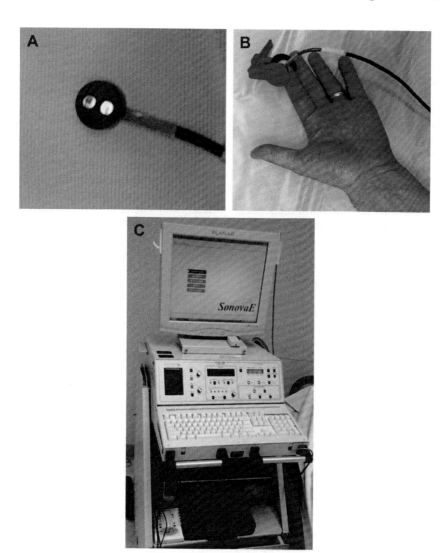

Fig. 9. Photoplethysmography is performed using a light-emitted diode (LED) sensor (*A*) that is placed on the examined digit (*B*). The signal is transmitted–received into computer software (*C*).

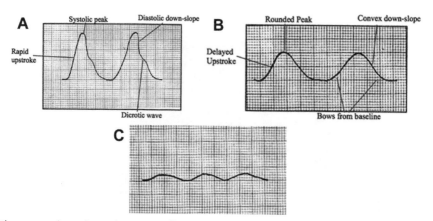

Fig. 10. Plethysmography pulse–volume recordings: normal (*A*), stenosis (*B*), occlusion (*C*).

recover from physiologic stress. The hand is submerged in water and exposed to 5°C to 8°C for approximately 3 to 5 minutes (**Fig. 11**).[1] By measuring digital temperature, the thermoregulatory ability of the vascular bed is evaluated. The test consists of 3 phases: a baseline phase with the hand at room temperature, a cooling phase with the hand exposed to cold temperatures, and a rewarming phase with the hand back at room temperature for about 20 minutes. Normal responses display temperature readings that parallel the curve for laser Doppler fluxometry. Abnormalities present as cold or warm responses. A cold response, often seen in women, is a decrease in digital temperature and microvascular perfusion when the hand is stressed to cold temperatures, whereas a warm response, seen twice as often in men as in women, is a sympathetic dysfunction in which few modulations in vascular tone occur. These response patterns help explain the pathogenesis of vascular occlusive syndromes, such as Raynaud phenomenon, occurring primarily in women.[8]

Direct examination of the nutritional papillary capillaries via the microscope is noninvasive, reproducible, and evaluates vascular problems of the upper extremity; however, the test is time consuming and technically challenging. Nail fold capillaroscopy visualizes capillary morphology for any structural changes and can quantify nutritional blood flow. Abnormal capillary morphology may lead to the diagnosis of systemic diseases.[1]

RADIOGRAPHIC STUDIES

Several tests are performed in the radiology suite to evaluate upper extremity tissue perfusion. Bone scan imaging has been used occasionally, most often in cases of frostbite. Angiography is the gold standard test to evaluate vascular pathology. Recently, noninvasive invasive tests such as computed tomography (CT) scanning and magnetic resonance imaging (MRI) with contrast dyes have provided detailed cross-sectional images of blood vessels and surrounding tissues.

Three-phase bone scan or scintigraphy is useful to demonstrate the extent of soft tissue damage and bone devitalization in cases of frostbite. Technetium-99m (Tc-99m) is a nuclear isomer that is taken up by osteoblasts, and so regions of active bone growth including bone tumors, metastasis, and fractures, are detected. There are 3 phases in scanning: flow phase, blood pool image, and delayed phase. The first phase detects perfusion of a lesion, as scans are obtained within seconds of Tc-99m injection. Blood pool images are obtained about 5 minutes after injection, evaluating the vascularity of the region. Finally, the delayed phase is performed about 3 hours after injection, such that most of the radioisotope has been metabolized, and so bone turnover associated with the lesion or region is assessed. Regarding the upper extremity, it has been most useful in evaluating patients with frostbite. Twomey and colleagues[9] studied 19 patients with frostbite and found that Tc-99m bone scanning was an accurate predictor of potential digital loss and level of digit amputation such that more invasive testing is unnecessary.

An angiogram (or arteriogram) is an invasive procedure that can be both diagnostic and therapeutic. After puncturing the arterial system and injecting a radio-opaque contrast agent, the blood vessels are visualized using fluoroscopy. Digital subtraction angiography (DSA), however, uses computer processing to manipulate the acquired data and subtract osseous structures or enhance vascular ones in real time (**Fig. 12**).[10] It can diagnose the cutoff level (**Fig. 13**) or segmental defect

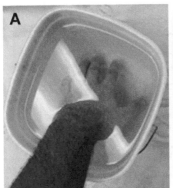 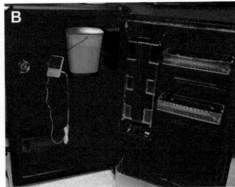

Fig. 11. Stress testing is performed by submerging the hand (*A*) in water cooled to 5°C to 8°C (40°F–50°F) (*B*).

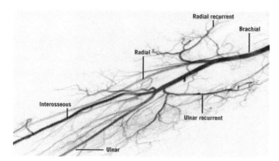

Fig. 12. Arterial anatomy of the forearm appreciated on digital subtraction angiography.

(**Fig. 14**). During this imaging, the interventional radiologist or vascular surgeon may attempt to dilate a lumen with balloon angioplasty, maintain vessel patency with a stent, or perform thrombolysis or thrombectomy for revascularization.[11] Nevertheless, the advancements of CT and magnetic resonance angiography have stimulated controversy regarding the necessity and timing of DSA.[12]

CT angiogram is comprised of high-resolution vascular images and cross-sectional slices of soft tissue structures adjacent to vascular ones such as bones and ligaments (**Fig. 15**). Iodine contrast dye must first be injected into the patient's venous system to achieve arterial enhancement. The radiation exposure of an upper extremity CT scan decreases from proximal to distal; the radiation dose is 2.06 mSv for the shoulder, 0.14 mSv for the elbow, and 0.03 mSv for the wrist. The complications from radiation exposure are small. Epidemiologic investigators have concluded that an acute exposure of 10 to 50 mSv may be potentially carcinogenic.[12] With the technological advances achieved to date, surrounding tissues are subtracted to isolate vascular structures. The rapid speed of image acquisition is vital in polytrauma patients.[13] CT angiogram is often performed before angiography when there is a high suspicion of arterial injury to become a road map for subsequent intervention (**Fig. 16**). It facilitates diagnosis in polytrauma patients in whom the osseous and soft tissue details are exceptional, and it aids in microsurgical reconstruction.[13,14]

Magnetic resonance arteriography (MRA) is combined with MRI to evaluate vascularity of the upper extremity in a noninvasive manner and eliminate the risks of radiation and renal failure or allergy associated with contrast dyes. MRA evaluates both the arterial and venous systems of the upper limb in a blood flow-dependent

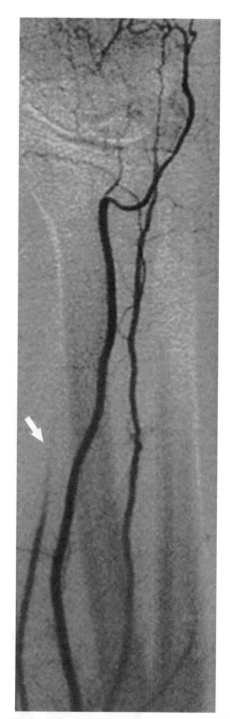

Fig. 13. Digital subtraction angiography visualizing radial artery cutoff (*arrow*).

manner while also evaluating adjacent soft tissue structures (**Fig. 17**).[15] The use of gadolinium–diethylenetriaminepentaacetic acid (Gd-DTPA) contrast in 3-dimensional pulse sequences enhances these multiangular projection images to

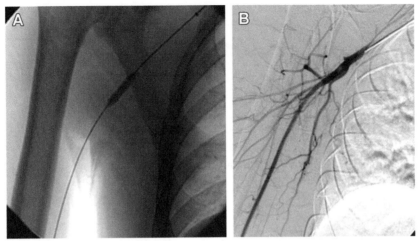

Fig. 14. Guide wire threading for dye injection (*A*). Once the dye is injected and fluoroscopy is performed, an axillary thrombus and intimal tear is visualized (*B*).

correlate obstruction or embolus with a physician's clinical suspicion of vascular compromise.[1,15] Gd-DTPA contrast elicits no allergic response and is typically injected in the contralateral antecubital vein. The part of the upper limb being imaged must be positioned appropriately in the gantry to ensure adequate coverage. For example, to image the hand and forearm, the patient is placed in a superman position (head toward gantry, shoulders fully flexed forward, and forearms pronated), while a patient with suspected thoracic outlet syndrome lies supine with the arm in the hyperabducted position.[16] MRA does have physical limitations. Maximum coverage is 40 to 50 cm, the contrast medium has variable circulation times, and overlap of the arteries and veins in the hand may make diagnosis difficult.

With the technological improvements of CT and MRI, noninvasive radiographic studies help examiners visualize vascular pathology in a noninvasive manner. Physical examination findings and physiologic control mechanisms are essential to establish vascular pathology and quantitate macro- and microvascular flow.[17]

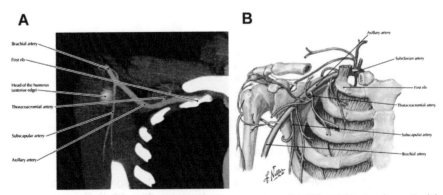

Fig. 15. CT angiography of a normal axillary artery (*A*) as compared to the Netter's schematic (*B*). (*From* [*A*] Weber EC, Vilensky JA, Carmichael SW, et al. Netter's concise radiologic anatomy. Philadelphia: Saunders; 2014, with permission; and [*B*] Netter illustration from www.netterimages.com. © Elsevier Inc. All rights reserved.)

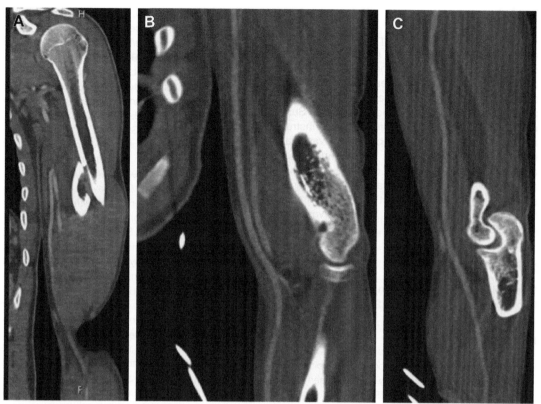

Fig. 16. CT angiogram of the left upper extremity demonstrating a midshaft humerus fracture and intact brachial artery medially (*A*). Imaging of the brachial artery becoming the radial (*B*) and ulnar (*C*) arteries. (*Courtesy of* C.C. Sexton, MD, Baltimore, MD.)

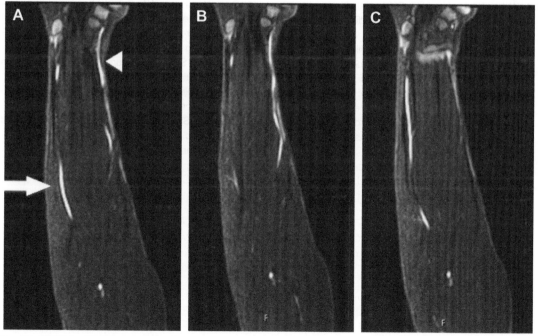

Fig. 17. Multiple slices from magnetic resonance angiography of the left forearm demonstrating (*A*) intact ulnar (*arrow*) and radial (*arrowhead*) arteries (*B*), continuation of radial artery, and (*C*) continuation of ulnar artery. (*Courtesy of* C.C. Sexton, MD, Baltimore, MD.)

SUMMARY

Vascular disorders of the upper limb can be devastating for a patient. The diagnosis of upper extremity vascular pathology includes noninvasive and invasive examinations. Treatment begins with a thorough patient interview and continues with pertinent physical examination findings. Suspected diagnoses can be confirmed using instruments available at the bedside, vascular laboratory, or radiology suite. With technological advances, radiographic tests continue to evolve and improve; however, evaluation of symptoms and their effect on the patient's daily life directs further diagnostic studies in both the vascular and radiology suites.

SUPPLEMENTARY DATA

Video related to this article can be found online at http://dx.doi.org/10.1016/j.hcl.2014.09.001.

REFERENCES

1. Chloros GD, Smerlis NN, Li Z, et al. Noninvasive evaluation of upper-extremity vascular perfusion. J Hand Surg Am 2008;33(4):591–600.

2. Thompson JC. Netter's concise orthopaedic anatomy. 2nd edition. Philadelphia: Saunders; 2010.

3. Gelberman RH, Blasingame JP. The timed Allen test. J Trauma 1981;21(6):477–9.

4. Weber TM, Lockhart ME, Robbin ML. Upper extremity venous Doppler ultrasound. Radiol Clin North Am 2007;45(3):513, ix.

5. Millet JD, Gunabushanam G, Ojili V, et al. Complications following vascular procedures in the upper extremities: a sonographic pictorial review. Ultrasound Q 2013;29(1):33–45.

6. Dumanian GA, Segalman K, Buehner JW, et al. Analysis of digital pulse-volume recordings with radial and ulnar artery compression. Plast Reconstr Surg 1998;102(6):1993–8.

7. Whiteley MS, Fox AD, Horrocks M. Photoplethysmography can replace hand-held Doppler in the measurement of ankle/brachial indices. Ann R Coll Surg Engl 1998;80(2):96–8.

8. Pollock FE Jr, Koman LA, Smith BP, et al. Measurement of hand microvascular blood flow with isolated cold stress testing and laser Doppler fluxmetry. J Hand Surg Am 1993;18(1):143–50.

9. Twomey JA, Peltier GL, Zera RT. An open-label study to evaluate the safety and efficacy of tissue plasminogen activator in treatment of severe frostbite. J Trauma 2005;59(6):1350–4.

10. Harrington DP, Boxt LM, Murray PD. Digital subtraction angiography: overview of technical principles. AJR Am J Roentgenol 1982;139(4):781–6.

11. Islam A, Edgerton C, Stafford JM, et al. Anatomic findings and outcomes associated with upper extremity arteriography and selective thrombolysis for acute finger ischemia. J Vasc Surg 2014;60(2):410–7.

12. Biswas D, Bible JE, Bohan M, et al. Radiation exposure from musculoskeletal computerized tomographic scans. J Bone Joint Surg Am 2009;91(8):1882–9.

13. Bozlar U, Ogur T, Norton PT, et al. CT angiography of the upper extremity arterial system: part 1—anatomy, technique, and use in trauma patients. AJR Am J Roentgenol 2013;201(4):745–52.

14. Bogdan MA, Klein MB, Rubin GD, et al. CT angiography in complex upper extremity reconstruction. J Hand Surg 2004;29B(5):465–9.

15. Disa JJ, CHung KC, Gellad FE, et al. Efficacy of magnetic resonance angiography in the evaluation of vascular malformations of the hand. Plast Reconstr Surg 1997;99(1):136–44.

16. Razek AA, Saad E, Soliman N, et al. Assessment of vascular disorders of the upper extremity with contrast-enhanced magnetic resonance angiography: pictorial review. Jpn J Radiol 2010;28(2):87–94.

17. Ruch DS, Smith TL, Smith BP, et al. Anatomic and physiologic evaluation of upper extremity ischemia. Microsurgery 1999;19(4):181–8.

The Role of Thrombolytics in Acute and Chronic Occlusion of the Hand

Randall R. De Martino, MD, MS[a],*, Steven L. Moran, MD[b]

KEYWORDS

- Hand ischemia • Thrombolytics • Thrombolysis • Catheter • Arterial occlusion

KEY POINTS

- Hand and digital artery thrombosis can be poorly tolerated if there is little collateral flow.
- Thrombolytic therapy is more favorable in the setting of acute thrombosis.
- Recombinant tissue plasminogen activator is the most common thrombolytic agent, and carries contraindications resulting from bleeding risks.
- Angiographic improvement should be expected in most cases of acute ischemia, and amputations are infrequent if no tissue necrosis is present.
- Attention to identification of serious hemorrhagic, thrombotic, and access-site complications is mandatory, as they are not uncommon.

INTRODUCTION

Hand ischemia represents a complex surgical problem for even the experienced clinician. The rarity of hand ischemia, the small caliber of the distal vasculature, and the limited surgical options available for treatment all compound the difficulty of intervention. Tissue necrosis and the need for amputation remain prevalent concerns in hand ischemia, even in the setting of prompt identification and treatment. This review discusses the role of thrombolytic therapy as an alternative or adjunctive therapeutic option for hand ischemia.

The upper extremity is less prone than the lower extremities to vascular compromise and limb-threatening ischemia, owing to the lower atherosclerotic disease burden seen in the upper extremities and the robust collateral blood supply. The hand is supplied by the continuation of the radial and ulnar arteries into the deep and superficial palmar arch collateral network that are dominated by radial and ulnar inflow, respectively (**Fig. 1**).[1] Distal to this, terminal common and proper digital vessels become end arteries with little ability to receive collateral flow. Although isolated radial or ulnar occlusion is well tolerated, occlusions more distal to this are poorly tolerated, and these occlusions are the focus of this article. Thrombosis and embolization to the palmar arch and digital arteries are prone to result in ischemic insults and tissue loss because of the end-organ nature of these vessels.

The natural history of hand and digital ischemia is difficult to describe because of the vast number of causes (acute and chronic) and tailored treatments for each. In addition, there is inconsistency in the literature regarding outcomes, making comparisons and description of outcomes difficult. In general, mild and moderate ischemia has a favorable prognosis, whereas severe ischemia, ulceration, and the presence of connective tissue

The authors have no relevant disclosures related to this work.
a Division of Vascular and Endovascular Surgery, Department of Surgery, Mayo Clinic, 200 First Street Southwest, Rochester, MN 55905, USA; b Division of Plastic Surgery, Department of Surgery, Mayo Clinic, 200 First Street Southwest, Rochester, MN 55905, USA
* Corresponding author.
E-mail address: demartino.randall@mayo.edu

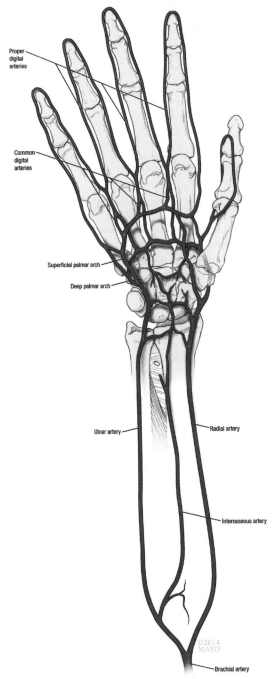

Proper
digital
arteries

Common
digital
arteries

Superficial palmar arch

Deep palmar arch

Ulnar artery

Radial artery

Interosseous artery

©2014
MAYO

Brachial artery

Fig. 1. Arterial anatomy of the hand. (*Courtesy of Mayo Foundation for Medical Education and Research, Rochester, MN, all rights reserved; with permission.*)

disease have higher rates of recurrent ulcers or need for amputation.[2]

ETIOLOGY

Upper extremity ischemia can be a result of numerous causes, and a description of all of these is outside the scope of this discussion. The etiology of more distal hand and digit ischemia, particularly those treated with thrombolysis, is more focused. The conditions listed in **Box 1** comprise the breadth of conditions encountered with hand ischemia. A good history and physical examination will help differentiate most of these. More narrowly, risk factors and causes for hand ischemia include smoking and atherosclerosis, connective tissue disease, occupational exposure to repetitive trauma, and hypercoagulable states.[3]

Differentiating between acute and chronic hand ischemia is important in planning for favorable outcomes to thrombolytic therapy. Situations of acute

---

Box 1
Causes of hand ischemia

Systemic

Atherosclerosis

Immune-mediated/inflammatory

- Scleroderma
- Rheumatoid arthritis
- Sjögren syndrome
- Systemic lupus erythematosus
- Hypersensitivity angiitis
- Henoch-Schönlein purpura
- Buerger disease

Myeloproliferative disorders

- Thrombocytosis
- Leukemia
- Polycythemia

Thrombotic

Hypercoagulable states

In situ thrombosis

Embolism

Traumatic

Iatrogenic injury

- Arterial catheterization
- Trauma
- Arterial drug injection

Cold injury

Vibration injury

Cytotoxic drugs

Other

Fibromuscular disease

Dialysis steal syndrome

vessel thrombosis are best suited for thrombolytic therapy; these typically present within several hours of onset, and are often due to in situ thrombosis or thrombosis from catheter-related access, embolism from a more central source, hypercoagulable states, and arterial drug injection. Many of the other causes listed in **Box 1** can result in more chronic arterial disease with damage to multiple arterial wall layers, which are unlikely to be successfully treated with thrombolysis.

THERAPEUTIC OPTIONS AND SURGICAL TECHNIQUE

The most important step in the management of any acutely ischemic limb is immediate anticoagulation (if possible) to limit subsequent thromboembolism, or progression of in situ thrombus. Therapeutic options for hand ischemia rely on removal of the offending thrombus within the vasculature and restoration of in-line perfusion to the digital arteries if possible. At this point, the treatment options for hand ischemia are often dictated by the disorder that has caused the ischemia. Embolism, in situ thrombosis, or a combination of the two represent most of the causes of hand ischemia, and the patient's history and physical examination will help identify these.

Hand ischemia from a proximal obstruction (such as an embolus in the brachial artery) and resulting from arterial disease of the proximal upper extremity and great vessels are not be discussed here. Often these conditions are treated with standard embolectomy or bypass techniques in addition to endovascular means. By contrast, occlusive ischemia of the hand and digits is difficult to treat with standard surgical approaches. In this setting, catheter-directed therapies such as intra-arterial thrombolysis have several advantages. First, arterial cannulation is done remotely, minimizing trauma to the vessels of interest. Modern low-profile catheter systems reduce the access size for treatment and reduce overall vessel trauma. Second, intra-arterial infusion of lytic agents can reduce the systemic effects of drug treatment and decrease the overall dose needed, reducing bleeding risk.

Contraindications

Thrombolytic drugs carry a risk of hemorrhagic complications (see later discussion). Absolute contraindications for thrombolytic therapy include active bleeding, uncontrolled clotting disorders, known intracranial neoplasm, and severe uncontrolled hypertension. Additional contraindications include recent (2 months) intracranial or spinal surgery, central nervous system trauma, and recent cerebrovascular accident. These situations carry an extremely high risk for intracranial or intraspinal bleed, or uncontrolled hemorrhage. Relative contraindications include recent (within prior 10 days) surgery, gastrointestinal bleed, or trauma. Pregnancy, acute pancreatitis, and advanced liver or kidney disease also merit additional concern for risk of significant bleeding. In addition, left heart thrombus may embolize with thrombolytic therapy. Careful judgment about the risk for other potential bleeding conditions is necessary before initiating treatment.

Thrombolytic Agents

Thrombolytic agents have evolved over the past 80 years. The first described agent was streptokinase, discovered in 1933 at Johns Hopkins University, although it was not used clinically until 1954. Streptokinase is a single-chain protein produced by B-hemolytic streptococci, and results in activation of plasminogen and initiation of the fibrinolytic cascade. Because of its bacterial origins, prior streptokinase administration or previous bacterial exposure can result in antibody formation, limiting its ability for repeated use.

Urokinase was approved for use in 1952 and overcame the antigenic limitation of streptokinase, as it is normally present in low concentrations in human plasma (urine-plasminogen activator) and works by cleaving plasminogen to plasmin. Although streptokinase and urokinase were the main thrombolytic agents for almost 50 years, neither agent is produced commercially in the United States today, although streptokinase remains available in other regions owing to its low cost.

At present, recombinant tissue plasminogen activator (rt-PA or alteplase) is the most commonly used thrombolytic drug, and is identical to naturally endogenous tissue plasminogen activator (t-PA) from endothelial cells. It has a short half-life of 5 minutes and currently is indicated for use in acute myocardial infarction, pulmonary embolism, central venous catheter occlusion, and acute stroke. It is also used in the setting of arterial and venous thrombosis. For catheter-directed extended infusions (>12 hours), typically 0.5 to 1 mg/h is infused into the target thrombus. Dosages up to 2.5 mg per hour may be possible, although increasing the dose also increases hemorrhagic risk. For short infusion durations (<12 hours) 0.05 mg/kg/h may be infused.

Technique

Diagnostic arteriography of the entire upper extremity should precede the initiation of thrombolytic therapy to help identify potential causes. This action can be taken by way of either a conventional catheter-based arteriogram of the arch and proximal upper extremity vessels, or a computed tomography (CT) arteriogram, depending on the quality of imaging available. For a conventional arteriogram, the femoral artery is the most common site of access (**Fig. 2**, lower inset). Fluoroscopy is used to identify the femoral head, and ultrasound is used to guide the femoral puncture and reduce the risk of inadvertent access of the external iliac or superficial femoral artery. Puncture of the external iliac or superficial femoral artery can result in significant bleeding complications in the setting of thrombolytic therapy. Access is obtained with a Micropuncture Access kit (Cook Medical, Bloomington, IN, USA) and upsized to a larger sheath using a standard Seldinger technique. Before traversing the aortic arch, heparin (100 U/kg) is administered. Arch aortography is then followed by catheterization of either the innominate artery or left subclavian artery, depending on the upper extremity of interest. Cannulation may be performed with a variety of specialized catheters. Once cannulated, dedicated arteriograms of the entire upper extremity should be done with superselective catheterization advanced to the brachial, radial, and ulnar arteries (see **Fig. 2**).

Once the decision for thrombolytic therapy has been made, the method of delivery for medication is determined. Thrombolytic therapy can be administered via either the femoral artery access already obtained or a separate antegrade puncture of the brachial artery (see **Fig. 2**, upper insert). The latter is more commonly reported in the literature, and may be preferable if aortography and proximal upper extremity arteriograms are not necessary. Brachial artery puncture makes access to the target lesions easier given its proximity to the hand and shorter working distance. In addition, depending on the patient's size, infusion catheter lengths may be limited to permit access from the groin down to the hand. The disadvantage of this approach is that the femoral access obtained may need to remain during thrombolytic treatment, as removal may result in bleeding during medication infusion.

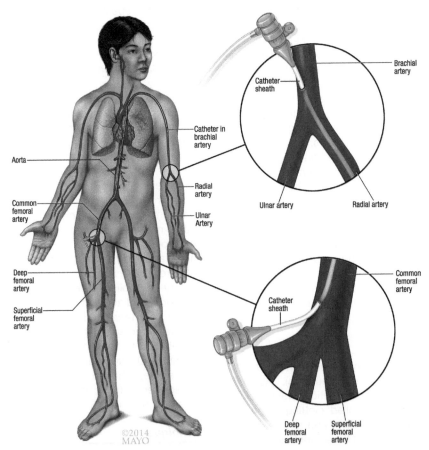

Fig. 2. Arterial access sites of the femoral and brachial arteries for intra-arterial thrombolytic treatment. (*Courtesy of* Mayo Foundation for Medical Education and Research, Rochester, MN, all rights reserved; with permission.)

Alternatively, the femoral artery access can be used for both the diagnostic and therapeutic treatment, which is achieved via selective catheterization from the groin to the hand (see **Fig. 2**, lower insert). The major drawback of this approach is the need for a catheter to lie across the vertebral artery origins. If the right arm is being treated, a catheter will sit across the carotid artery origins in the aortic arch for an extended period of time, which may result in thrombus formation and a potential risk of embolic stroke. The optimal approach would include a CT arteriogram of the great vessels, followed by a single brachial access approach for thrombolytic treatment.

Regardless of access location, typical arterial access is secured with a 4F or 5F sheath. For brachial access, a smaller (4F) sheath is preferable (see **Fig. 2**). Infusion of vasodilators may be necessary, as arterial spasm is common during manipulation of arteries to the upper extremity, and is treated with intra-arterial injection of nitroglycerine or verapamil. Standard guide wires are used to navigate to the vessel of interest, and preferably into the thrombus. Once in this location, a lytic infusion catheter (Cragg-McNamara; Covidien, Plymouth, MN, USA; or UniFuse; Angiodynamics, Lytham, NY, USA) can be advanced over the wire. These catheters have multiple side holes over a variable treatment length (5–50 cm) for intrathrombus infusion (**Fig. 3**). These catheters typically permit placement of an infusion wire through the hole at the distal end to permit infusion distal to the thrombus (Katzen wire; Boston Scientific, Natick, MA, USA; or ProStream; Covidien). Although adjuncts exist to assist thrombolytic treatment (mechanical maceration or ultrasonography), these have little role in the treatment of very distal end arteries such as those of the hand.

Once the catheter has been placed within the thrombus, or as close to it as possible, 1 to 2 mg t-PA may be infused to prime the catheter.

A continuous pump is then used to infuse for ongoing treatment, typically at a rate of 0.5 to 1 mg/h (**Fig. 4**). In addition, unfractionated heparin is infused through the access sheath to minimize the risk of perisheath thrombus formation (500 U/h). The patient is then placed in a monitored setting, such as the intensive care unit, for observation during treatment. It is crucial that the patient is continually assessed for signs of bleeding, both at the access site and remote sites. In addition, routine blood work is performed, including blood counts, prothrombin time, partial thromboplastin time, international normalized ratio, and fibrinogen levels, every 4 to 6 hours. A decrease in the fibrinogen level may indicate systemic release of the drug with systemic fibrinolysis. The authors' institutional practice is to halve the t-PA dose for a fibrinogen level that drops to less than 200 mg/dL, and cease administration for values less than 100 mg/dL.

Reassessment for angiographic and clinical improvement is necessary during treatment. Repeat arteriograms (lytic checks) are performed between 12 and 24 hours after the initiation of treatment, or from the last lytic check. Treatment can safely be administered for 24 to 48 hours. Longer treatments are possible, although the bleeding risks increase with longer treatment duration. In addition, residual thrombus that remains after 48 hours may represent more organized chronic thrombus with a lower likelihood of successful lysis.

Once the decision to cease treatment has been made, typically the catheter can be pulled safely 1 hour after the infusion has been stopped, owing to the short half-life of t-PA. Heparin should be flushed through the sheath while waiting for removal to minimize perisheath thrombus formation. Manual pressure is held over the access site for hemostasis. Therapeutic anticoagulation can be resumed shortly after sheath removal.

CLINICAL OUTCOMES

Since the original description of intra-arterial thrombolytic therapy by Dotter and colleagues[4] in 1974, scattered case reports and series have been reported over the past 40 years. Reported series range from 1 to 16 patients being treated for distal arm and hand arterial occlusive disease with thrombolytic therapy.[3–22] Objective description of the level of ischemia, original and completion angiographic findings, and long-term clinical outcomes are variable, making firm conclusions difficult.

Although Dotter's original series had only 2 patients with distal arm ischemia, neither of whom

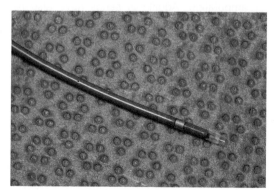

Fig. 3. Cragg-McNamara thrombolytic catheter. (*Courtesy of* Covidien, Plymouth, MN; with permission.)

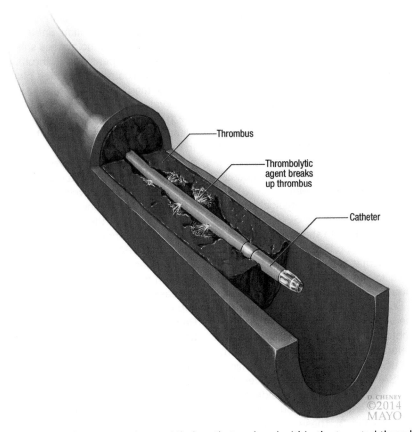

Thrombus

Thrombolytic agent breaks up thrombus

Catheter

D. CHENEY
©2014
MAYO

Fig. 4. Infusion of thrombolytic agents via a multihole catheter placed within the targeted thrombus for continuous infusion. (*Courtesy of* Mayo Foundation for Medical Education and Research, Rochester, MN, all rights reserved; with permission.)

improved with thrombolytic therapy, successful reports have been described since that time. Overall, angiographic or clinical improvement is reported to occur nearly 80% of the time. Fortunately, the incidence of amputation appears to be less than 10%. These amputations are often at the digital level, and the hand is often spared even with only partial recanalization. The most consistently successful reported cases (angiographic resolution of thrombus) involved acute presentation of hand ischemia with prompt treatment. Cases reporting patients with chronic thrombus (greater than 1–2 weeks) appear to have less favorable results. Most cases of chronic thrombus show no improvement or only partial recanalization.[13,19] This finding is intuitive, as mature thrombus is typically less amenable to thrombolysis. For thrombolytic therapy for venous or lower extremity arterial indications, thrombus present for more than 2 weeks is typically not considered for treatment for this reason.

Embolism arising from cardiogenic sources, such as atrial fibrillation, is often thought to contain mature thrombus that is not amenable to thrombolysis. Nevertheless, successful reports of catheter-directed thrombolysis for such conditions exist. Miyayama and colleagues[18] reported a series of 4 patients with hand ischemia from presumed atrial fibrillation, all of whom were treated with urokinase. Half had complete thrombus resolution and half had a partial response, with no need for amputation. Additional series have also reported successful attempts in this setting.[9,21] Potentially, patients with new-onset atrial fibrillation may be the best candidates in this setting, as the thrombus is more likely to be acute.

Thrombolysis is often used for hypothenar hammer syndrome if ulnar artery thrombosis occurs with distal embolization, often as an adjunct to subsequent arterial reconstruction. In one series after thrombolysis, bypass was required in 1 of 4 patients and partial finger amputations in a second patient.[21] The remaining patients did not undergo further intervention. However, in series of 7 patients with radiographic follow-up after thrombolytic therapy alone for hypothenar hammer syndrome, 43% had progression of their arterial occlusive disease and only 29% remained stable, supporting the need for surgical repair for this specific disorder.[10]

Thrombolysis in the setting of intra-arterial drug injections has mixed results. Some series have reported complete angiographic improvement without the need for amputation,[6,7,12] whereas other reports resulted in no improvement and/or digital amputation.[4,5,8] Treatment of radial artery thrombosis from invasive arterial line placement has been successful, with no need for subsequent intervention.[11] However, treatment is unlikely to be successful once the thrombus is chronic.[20] Treatment of Buerger disease with thrombolytic therapy is rarely reported. The only dedicated report demonstrated favorable results with complete recanalization of the occluded vessels (**Fig. 5**).[17] Remaining causes, such as in situ thrombosis, atheroembolism, polycythemia vera, systemic lupus erythematosus, and cryptogenic sources, have been treated with variable success. Given the few patients reported, conclusions are difficult. Results appear similar to those for other malignancies, with favorable results in the acute setting.

Patients who present with profound tissue ischemia or necrosis appear to be at high risk for amputation.[14] Nevertheless, a review of a 34 upper extremity thrombolytic cases (16 of which included the distal arm and hand) demonstrated that thrombolytic therapy for these patients has a trend toward improved amputation-free survival in comparison with conservative management alone. This finding suggests that despite advanced ischemia, thrombolytic treatment may be reasonable in this setting to reduce the risk of amputation.[3]

COMPLICATIONS AND CONCERNS

Overall complication rates of reported studies for upper extremity thrombolytic therapy range from 0% to 75% of patients treated. Nearly half of the reported cases have no complications, but the remaining series report an 11% to 75% complication rate (for a pooled complication rate of 18%). The most common complication is bleeding, which results from percutaneous arterial access to the femoral or brachial artery and the use of a thrombolytic agent. Bleeding may occur at the access site, or remotely (intracranial hemorrhage, visceral or retroperitoneal hematoma). Major bleeding (disability or need for transfusion) has been reported for other thrombolytic indications (eg, myocardial infarction, pulmonary embolism, stroke) to range from 1% to 30% of patients. Intracranial hemorrhage has been reported to be as high as 8% for acute ischemic stroke, but typically is much lower (1%) for catheter-directed treatment.[23] Overall bleeding rate (major and minor) for upper extremity thrombolysis reported in the literature is approximately 8%. There have been no reports of intracranial hemorrhage in this setting, but transient ischemic attacks have been reported.[9,16] In addition to bleeding, thrombotic complications such as catheter-related thrombus formation and embolization could result is distal arterial bed ischemia, and has been reported during upper extremity thrombolysis.[16,22] Finally, removal of the sheath while on anticoagulation can result in pseudoaneurysm formation.

Patients need to be monitored closely for these complications. Access-site bleeding, limb swelling, abdominal or back pain, or altered mental status should alert the clinician to a potential bleeding complication. If bleeding is

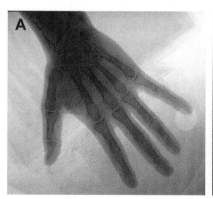
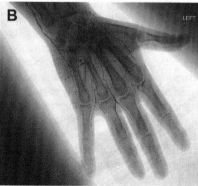

Fig. 5. Angiographic images of a 46-year-old man with history of suspected Buerger disease. The patient presented with symptoms of finger ischemia of several weeks' duration. (*A*) Prethrombolysis angiogram shows minimal filling of digital vessels. (*B*) Following 24 hours of tissue plasminogen activator therapy there is improvement in the flow through the hand, as seen in filling of the digital vessels.

suspected, thrombolytic therapy should be stopped immediately and appropriate imaging performed (head, abdomen, or pelvis CT as indicated). Often bleeding will stop with cessation of thrombolytic or anticoagulation treatment. Full correction of anticoagulation may be required. Surgical decompression or embolization of bleeding branches may be necessary. Decompression is mandatory for brachial access-site hematomas, owing to median nerve compression. Moreover, muscular hematomas in distal upper extremity may require fasciotomy if they result in compartment syndrome.[8]

Other less common complications include fever, fluid overload, skin necrosis, transfusion reactions, contrast reaction or nephropathy, catheter-related sepsis, and antigenic response (if streptokinase is used). A review of complications for thrombolytic therapy demonstrated that complications occur in the setting of bleeding mismanagement, poor patient selection, and protocol breaches. Bleeding may be mismanaged by delays in recognition, failure to appropriately decompress hematomas, or failure to recognize subtle signs of intracranial bleeding (such as headache). Patients with a recent surgery or procedures, limb ischemia resulting from trauma, or non–limb-threatening ischemia may be at high risk for complications. Finally, overzealous heparinization, prolonged treatment (>48 hours), and adjustment of thrombolytic dosage outside of institutional protocols also place patients at risk for bleeding complications.[24] Overall, clinicians must be diligent in monitoring patients for complications while undergoing thrombolytic therapy, and should have the resources available to manage these complications as they are not uncommon.

SUMMARY

Catheter-directed thrombolytic therapy is a useful therapeutic option in the setting of severe hand and digital ischemia. Overall, favorable results should be expected, particularly when thrombolysis is performed in the acute setting. Thrombolytic therapy performed for chronic thrombus appears to have much less benefit and is unlikely to be successful for thrombus that is present for more than 2 weeks. A thorough evaluation to find the cause of hand ischemia is necessary to prevent recurrence and ensure the best functional outcome for the hand. Following thrombolytic therapy amputation seems to be infrequent, and patients presenting with ongoing tissue loss from hand ischemia are at the highest risk for subsequent amputation. However, this should not dissuade the provider from considering thrombolytic therapy to salvage as much tissue as possible. Thrombolytic agents carry a high-risk profile, and bleeding complications are common. A careful evaluation of the risks weighed against the anticipated benefit is necessary. When therapy is under way, diligent monitoring is necessary to ensure optimal outcomes.

REFERENCES

1. Valentine RJ, Wind GG. Anatomic exposures in vascular surgery. 2nd edition. Philadelphia: Lippincott Williams & Wilkins; 2003.
2. McLafferty RB, Edwards JM, Taylor LM Jr, et al. Diagnosis and long-term clinical outcome in patients diagnosed with hand ischemia. J Vasc Surg 1995; 22(4):361–7 [discussion: 367–9].
3. Islam A, Edgerton C, Stafford JM, et al. Anatomic findings and outcomes associated with upper extremity arteriography and selective thrombolysis for acute finger ischemia. J Vasc Surg 2014;60(2):410–7.
4. Dotter CT, Rosch J, Seaman AJ. Selective clot lysis with low-dose streptokinase. Radiology 1974; 111(1):31–7.
5. Andreev A, Kavrakov T, Petkov D, et al. Severe acute hand ischemia following an accidental intraarterial drug injection, successfully treated with thrombolysis and intraarterial Iloprost infusion. Case report. Angiology 1995;46(10):963–7.
6. Barbiero G, Cognolato D, Casarin A, et al. Intra-arterial thrombolysis of acute hand ischaemia with or without microcatheter: preliminary experience and comparison with the literature. Radiol Med 2011; 116(6):919–31.
7. Bounameaux H, Schneider PA, Huber-Sauteur E, et al. Severe ischemia of the hand following intraarterial promazine injection: effects of vasodilation, anticoagulation, and local thrombolysis with tissue-type plasminogen activator. Vasa 1990;19(1):68–71.
8. Breguet R, Terraz S, Righini M, et al. Acute hand ischemia after unintentional intraarterial injection of drugs: is catheter-directed thrombolysis useful? J Vasc Interv Radiol 2014;25(6):963–8.
9. Coulon M, Goffette P, Dondelinger RF. Local thrombolytic infusion in arterial ischemia of the upper limb: mid-term results. Cardiovasc Intervent Radiol 1994;17(2):81–6.
10. Friedrich KM, Fruhwald-Pallamar J, Stadlbauer A, et al. Hypothenar hammer syndrome: long-term follow-up of selective thrombolysis by 3.0-T MR angiography. Eur J Radiol 2010;75(2):e27–31.
11. Geschwind JF, Dagli MS, Lambert DL, et al. Thrombolytic therapy in the setting of arterial line-induced ischemia. J Endovasc Ther 2003;10(3):590–4.
12. Ipaktchi K, Ipaktchi R, Niederbichler AD, et al. Unrecognized hand ischemia after intraarterial drug injection: successful management of a "near miss" event. Patient Saf Surg 2008;2(1):32.

13. Jelalian C, Mehrhof A, Cohen IK, et al. Streptokinase in the treatment of acute arterial occlusion of the hand. J Hand Surg 1985;10(4):534–8.

14. Johnson SP, Durham JD, Subber SW, et al. Acute arterial occlusions of the small vessels of the hand and forearm: treatment with regional urokinase therapy. J Vasc Interv Radiol 1999;10(7):869–76.

15. Kartchner MM, Wilcox WC. Thrombolysis of palmar and digital arterial thrombosis by intra-arterial thrombolysin. J Hand Surg 1976;1(1):67–74.

16. Lambiase RE, Paolella LP, Haas RA, et al. Extensive thromboembolic disease of the hand and forearm: treatment with thrombolytic therapy. J Vasc Interv Radiol 1991;2(2):201–8.

17. Lang EV, Bookstein JJ. Accelerated thrombolysis and angioplasty for hand ischemia in Buerger's disease. Cardiovasc Intervent Radiol 1989;12(2):95–7.

18. Miyayama S, Yamashiro M, Shibata Y, et al. Thrombolysis and thromboaspiration for acute thromboembolic occlusion in the upper extremity. Jpn J Radiol 2012;30(2):180–4.

19. Sullivan KL, Minken SL, White RI Jr. Treatment of a case of thromboembolism resulting from thoracic outlet syndrome with intra-arterial urokinase infusion. J Vasc Surg 1988;7(4):568–71.

20. Tisnado J, Bartol DT, Cho SR, et al. Low-dose fibrinolytic therapy in hand ischemia. Radiology 1984; 150(2):375–82.

21. Wheatley MJ, Marx MV. The use of intra-arterial urokinase in the management of hand ischemia secondary to palmar and digital arterial occlusion. Ann Plast Surg 1996;37(4):356–62 [discussion: 362–53].

22. Widlus DM, Venbrux AC, Benenati JF, et al. Fibrinolytic therapy for upper-extremity arterial occlusions. Radiology 1990;175(2):393–9.

23. Cronenwett JL, Johnston KW. Rutherford's vascular surgery. 8th edition. Philadelphia: Saunders/Elsevier; 2014.

24. Hirshberg A, Schneiderman J, Garniek A, et al. Errors and pitfalls in intraarterial thrombolytic therapy. J Vasc Surg 1989;10(6):612–6.

The Role of Botulinum Toxin in Vasospastic Disorders of the Hand

Michael W. Neumeister, MD, FRCSC, FACS

KEYWORDS

- Vasospasm • Raynaud • Botox • Botulinum toxin • Vasodilation • Pain • Ischemia

KEY POINTS

- At present, botulinum injections offer a low-risk method for the treatment of symptomatic Raynaud phenomenon.
- Although the mechanism has not been fully elucidated, this finding provides patients with another means of medical management before moving to sympathectomy.
- Repeated injections may be required.

INTRODUCTION

The hand is a true end organ with an arborization of vasculature that continues from the palms to the fingertips and nail beds. A multitude of intrinsic and extrinsic factors can affect the normal anatomy and physiology of the blood vessels to the hand. Blood vessels may be affected by trauma, inflammation, infection, autoimmune disorders, pharmacologic agents, neoplasms, and endocrine abnormalities, as well as other factors that may affect the central nervous system, the peripheral nervous system, and the neuropeptides that control vascular tone. Vasospasm, which is defined as inappropriate tone of the arteries or veins in the hand, can result in impaired vasodilatation, cold intolerance, and digital ischemia. It is estimated that more than 9 million people have vasospasm of the digits annually.[1-4] Women are more susceptible than men at a ratio of 9:1 and young adults experience more vasospastic episodes that those more than 40 years of age.[1-4] Although advances have been made in the last decade, understanding of digital vasospasm, also known as Raynaud phenomenon, is still limited. This article focuses on vasospasm of the hand and the use

of botulinum toxin for the treatment of patients with Raynaud phenomenon.

VASCULAR INSUFFICIENCY FROM VASOSPASM OF THE DIGITAL VESSELS

Vasospastic disorders of the hand are a common phenomenon and are manifest by remitting and relapsing clinical symptoms. Recurring episodes of vasospasm become problematic as the frequency and duration of the episodes increase. One of the earliest descriptions of vasospasm of digital arteries was by Maurice Raynaud in 1862, who described the process as "A local asphyxia of the extremities as the result of increased irritability of the central parts of the cord presiding over vascular innervation."[5,6] The vasospastic disorder characterized by Maurice Raynaud was called Raynaud disease for decades until John Hutchinson in 1901 correctly articulated that there were many causes for vasospasm of the digital vessels and that the term "disease" was probably not appropriate for this condition. Sir Thomas Louis was the first to describe the physiologic features to distinguish primary Raynaud phenomenon from secondary Raynaud conditions.[5] Primary

The author is a consultant for MTF.

Institute for Plastic Surgery, Southern Illinois University School of Medicine, 747 North Rutledge, 3rd Floor, PO Box 19653, Springfield, IL 62794, USA

E-mail address: mneumeister@siumed.edu

Hand Clin 31 (2015) 23–37
http://dx.doi.org/10.1016/j.hcl.2014.09.003
0749-0712/15/$ – see front matter © 2015 Elsevier Inc. All rights reserved.

Box 1
Conditions associated with secondary Raynaud

Rheumatologic disease

  Systemic sclerosis

  Systemic lupus erythematosus

  Mixed connective tissue disease

  Dermatomyositis

  Rheumatoid arthritis

  Sjögren syndrome

  Vasculitis

Vascular occlusive disease

  Buerger disease

  Arteriosclerosis

  Thromboembolic disease

Drug induced

  Amphetamines

  Beta-adrenergic blockers

  Bleomycin

  Cisplatin

  Cyclosporin

  Ergots

  Interferon alfa

  Vinblastine

Hematologic syndromes

  Polycythemia

  Paraproteinemia

  Cryoglobulinemia

  Cryofibrinogenemia

  Cold agglutinin disease

  Homocysteinemia

  Protein C, protein S, antithrombin III deficiency

  Factor V Leiden

Environmental associations

  Vibration injury

  Frostbite

Anatomic syndromes

  Scalenus anticus syndrome

  Cervical rib

Infectious causes

  Hepatitis B and C (associated with cryoglobulinemia)

  Mycoplasma infections (cold agglutinins)

  Parvovirus B19

Many medical conditions or illnesses may have one of their manifestations present as Raynaud. The many potential causes or related entities that are associated with secondary Raynaud phenomenon are indicated here.

Adapted from Bakst R, Merola JF, Franks AG Jr, et al. Raynaud's phenomenon: pathogenesis and management. J Am Acad Dermatol 2008;59(4):635; with permission.

Raynaud phenomenon does not have any other associated medical condition linked to the vasospastic disorder. In secondary Raynaud phenomenon, the vasospastic disorder is linked to other systemic disorders (**Box 1, Table 1**).[1,6]

The term Raynaud phenomenon is used here to describe the clinical picture of pallor, cyanosis, and rubor. The disorder is the result of vascular embarrassment to the hand from dysfunction of the homeostatic neural control of blood vessels. The resultant paroxysmal vasoconstriction combined with episodes of vasodilation manifest in the color changes noted earlier, pain, and ultimately ulceration of the fingertips. The histories obtained from patients often describe their fingers as being blanched and cool, which is especially brought on by cold exposure or stress (**Fig. 1**). There are episodes of secondary vasodilation in which the digit becomes more swollen and fusiform with characteristic dysesthesias. The longer and more severe the vasospasm, the more likely the patient is to experience fingertip pain and possible ulceration. Persistent ischemia may lead to deep ulceration, bone exposure, and amputation.[7,8]

The physical examination findings on patients with Raynaud disease or phenomenon may appear normal when a vasospastic episode has not occurred recently. The surgeon should look for signs of ulceration, inflammation, dry gangrene, discoloration, nail bed petechiae, poor turgor, or dystrophic nails or fingertips. The capillary refill may be normal or sluggish but the Allen test is usually normal.

Tests used to evaluate the vascularity of the hand are included in **Box 2**. The management of Raynaud phenomenon is variable depending on the cause and the severity of the condition. Essential conservative measures include smoking cessation, maintaining a warm environment, and reducing stress. These early measures are often enough for those patients who have mild or very infrequent bouts of vasoconstriction. When vasospastic disorders result in prolonged symptomatic problems for patients, drug therapy is indicated. An extensive array of medications has been used

Table 1
Different characteristics of primary versus secondary Raynaud phenomenon

Characteristics	Primary	Secondary
Associated autoimmune disease	No	Yes
Age at onset (y)	<30	>30
Pain with attacks	Infrequent	Frequent
Finger involvement	Symmetric	Asymmetrical
Nail fold capillaries	Normal	Dilated with vessel dropout
Onycholysis and/or pterygium inversum	Infrequent	Frequent
Tuft pits and/or necrosis	Infrequent	Frequent
Autoantibodies	Negative or low titers	Increased titers

Primary Raynaud phenomenon is not associated with any condition. Secondary Raynaud phenomenon is related to other conditions or diseases.

Adapted from Bakst R, Merola JF, Franks AG Jr, et al. Raynaud's phenomenon: pathogenesis and management. J Am Acad Dermatol 2008;59(4):635; with permission.

Box. 2
Tests used to evaluate perfusion in the hand

Doppler

Doppler ultrasonography

Digital plethysmography (pulse volume recordings)

Radial-brachial index = 1.0

Digital-brachial index = 1.0

Less than 0.7 is abnormal, compromising healing of ulcers, wounds

Less than 0.5 indicates impending cell death (hand or digital ischemia)

From 0.7 to 1.0 indicates arterial flow compromise

Color duplex imaging

Oxygen saturation

Greater than 90% on room air; compare with contralateral side

Skin surface temperature determination ($\sim 30^{\circ}$C)

Laser Doppler fluxmetry

Cold stress testing

Hands exposed to cool air or water (5–8°C)

Laser Doppler perfusion imaging

Vital capillaroscopy

Scintigraphy

Magnetic resonance angiography

Computed tomography angiography

Many investigations can be used to help define normal and abnormal vascularity and perfusion of the digits.

for vasospastic disorders. Each medication has been used to block a certain part of the chain of events thought to be involved with vasospasm of the digital vessels. **Box 3** lists the mediators of vascular tone in the hand. The first-line drug used in Raynaud phenomenon is usually a calcium channel blocker to induce vasodilation of the digital vessels.[1,6,9–35] **Table 2** shows the various pharmacologic treatments to manage Raynaud phenomenon.[36–40] Many medications have been tried for this problematic disorder, which indicates that there is no gold standard or so-called magic bullet for the treatment of vasospasm in the hand. Many studies have shown some benefit with the use of these medications, although recalcitrant vasospasm still occurs in many patients, especially those with secondary Raynaud phenomenon.[1,41] Recent, promising studies have focused on phosphodiesterase 5 (PDE 5) inhibitors as a potential oral treatment of Raynaud.[42–50] Lin and colleagues[51] reviewed the role of PDE 5 in vascular homeostasis. They noted that the human

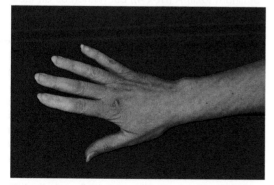

Fig. 1. Raynaud phenomenon characterized by digital ischemia, pain, and occasional ulcerations.

Box 3
Mediators of the vascular tone of the hand

- Sympathetic nervous system
  - Alpha adrenergic receptors of smooth muscle (alpha 2c)
    - Norepinephrine
- Parasympathetic nervous system
- Central nervous system
- Nitric oxide/cyclic GMP system
- Reactive oxygen species
- Redox pathways
- Rho kinase
- Estrogen
- Substance-P
- Calcitonin gene–related peptide
- Neuropeptide Y
- Vasoactive intestinal peptide
- Glutamate
- Prostacyclin (prostaglandin I2)
- Endothelium-derived hyperpolarizing factor
- Endothelium 1
- Thromboxane
- Angiotensin
- Platelet activation

The vessels of the hand and digits respond to stimuli from various sources, including nerve endings, humoral factors, tissue activation, and intrinsic factors. The multifactorial influence signals the balance of vasoconstriction and vasodilation.

genome encodes 21 phosphodiesterase genes. Furthermore the genes could be grouped into 11 families with almost 100 isoforms. PDE 5 and its 3 isoforms A1, A2, and A3 are the most studied phosphodiesterase enzymes that play a role in peripheral vascular control.

PDE 5 is affects vasodilatation through its effects on guanosine monophosphate (GMP) and the nitric oxide cycle. Nitric oxide, a natural vasodilator, has 3 isoforms of nitric oxide synthase: inducible nitric oxide synthase, endothelial nitric oxide synthase, and neural nitric oxide synthase. Nitric oxide activates guanylate cyclase to increase cyclic GMP levels, which induce smooth muscle relaxation ultimately producing vasodilation of blood vessels. Pathologic imbalance of nitric oxide levels may influence the normal physiologic regulation of vascular tone in the digits.

PDE 5 degrades cyclic GMP and therefore limits vasodilation within the physiologic norm. PDE 5 inhibitors prevent the degradation of cyclic GMP to promote long-lasting vasodilatation of vessels. Although most commonly used for erectile dysfunction, PDE 5 inhibitors are being used for other vascular disorders including Raynaud phenomenon. Numerous case reports (level V evidence) and case series (level IV evidence) have shown improvements with respect to the number and severity of the spastic attacks in patients treated with PDE 5 inhibitors, but 2 of 3 randomized, controlled, double-blinded studies (level II evidence) have failed to show any significant benefit.[42,50,52–54]

BOTULINUM TOXIN

In 1897, Emile van Ermengen, a microbiologist at the University of Ghent, Belgium, discovered that the bacterium *Clostridium botulinum* was responsible for producing the protein botulinum toxin.[5] *C botulinum* is a gram-negative, spore-forming, obligate anaerobic bacterium and is considered one of nature's most potent neuroparalytic agents. P. Tessmer Snipe and Hermann Sommer first purified the toxin in 1928.[55] The first elucidation of the mechanism of action of botulinum toxin as an inhibitor of acetylcholine release at neuromuscular junctions was described in 1949 by Arnold Burgen.[56] There are 8 serologically different types of botulinum toxin (A–H). The protein consists of a light chain (50 kDa) and a heavy chain (100 kDa) joined by a disulfide bond.[57] Botulinum toxin is considered one of the most lethal toxins known, with a median lethal dose of 1.3 to 2.1 ng/kg when administered intravenously or intramuscularly. One gram of botulinum toxin has the potential to kill 1 million people. However, in limited doses, botulinum toxin A and B have been used for therapeutic reasons. The US Food and Drug Administration (FDA) has approved 8 different uses for botulinum toxin A (**Box 4**), but numerous off-label uses have been documented in the literature as well (**Box 5**).[57,58]

Botulinum toxin's most commonly known mechanism of action is at the nerve ends of the neuromuscular junction.[59] The toxin is taken up by the nerve endings. The light chain of the toxin is an enzyme that cleaves a membrane-bound protein, called synaptosomal-associated protein 25 (SNAP-25), on the acetylcholine-filled vesicles. This cleavage prevents transport and exocytosis of the acetylcholine. The inhibition of acetylcholine release across the neuromuscular junction prevents muscle contraction, clinically manifesting as paralysis. However, the clinical manifestations

Table 2
Pharmacologic treatment of Raynaud phenomenon

Medication	Dosage	Comments
Calcium Channel Blockers		
Nifedipine	10–30 mg TID	Least cardioselective, most efficacious class
Nifedipine, sustained release	30–90 mg QD	Sustained release preparation reduces side effects
Felodipine	2.5–10 mg QD	—
Amlodipine	2.5–10 mg QD	—
Diltiazem, sustained release	120–33 mg QD	Intermediate cardioselectivity, minimal controlled data
Verapamil	40–120 mg TID	Most cardioselective, benefit not shown
Vasodilators		
Nitroglycerin	0.25–0.5 in topical 1%	Benefit shown; significant side effects avoided
Nitroglycerin	0.25–0.5 in topical 2%	Significant side effects from systemic absorption
L-Arginine	2–8 g QD	Useful in patients with low blood pressure
Sodium nitroprusside	0.3 μg/kg/min/IV	Used in critical ischemia
Prostaglandins		
Intravenous iloprost	0.5–2.0 ng/kg/min IV for 1–5 d	Used in critical ischemia
Oral iloprost	50–100 μg BID	Conflicting data regarding oral prostaglandins
Beraprost	60 μg TID	Conflicting data regarding oral prostaglandins
Epoprostenol	0.5–6 ng/kg/min for 2–5 d	Used in critical ischemia
Phosphodiesterase Inhibitors		
Sildenafil	50 mg BID	One placebo-controlled trial indicated benefit
Cilostazol	50–100 mg BID	One placebo-controlled trial indicated benefit
ACE Inhibitors		
Enalapril	2.5–20 mg QD	Few controlled data
Captopril	6.5–25 mg TID	Few controlled data
Losartan	50 mg QD	One placebo-controlled trial indicated benefit
Selective Serotonin Reuptake Inhibitors		
Fluoxetine	20 mg QD	One pilot study indicated benefit
Endothelin Receptor Antagonists		
Bosentan	62.5–125 mg BID	Reduces number of new ulcers but no benefit shown compared with existing ones; hepatotoxic

(*continued on next page*)

Table 2
(*continued*)

Medication	Dosage	Comments
Sympatholytics		
Prazosin	1–5 mg BID	Efficacy transient, may wane over time
Guanethidine	10–50 mg QD	Few controlled data
Phenoxybenzamine	10 mg QID	Few controlled data
Rho Kinase Inhibition		
Fasudil	30 mg/min for 30 min IV	Benefit shown in treatment of severe pulmonary hypertension
Anticoagulation/Antithrombotic		
Low-molecular-weight heparin	—	Used in critical ischemia
Warfarin	—	Few controlled data
Aspirin	81–325 mg QD	Few controlled data
Dipyridamole	75–100 mg QID	Few controlled data
Tissue plasminogen activator	—	Used in critical ischemia
Antioxidants		
Probucol	500 mg QD	Few controlled data
Botulinum toxin	40–100 U/hand	Improve perfusion, decrease pain
Miscellaneous		
Vitamin E	500 U QD	Useful in patients with low blood pressure
Slo-Niacin	250 mg QD	Useful in patients with low blood pressure
Griseofulvin (microsize)	500 mg daily	Useful in patients with low blood pressure
Pentoxifylline	400 mg TID	Useful in patients with low blood pressure

Many drugs have been used to treat Raynaud to inhibit vasospasm and improve blood flow.

Abbreviations: ACE, angiotensin-converting enzyme; BID, twice a day; IV, intravenous; QD, daily; QID, 4 times a day; TID, 3 times a day.

Adapted from Bakst R, Merola JF, Franks AG Jr, et al. Raynaud's phenomenon: pathogenesis and management. J Am Acad Dermatol 2008;59(4):643; with permission.

Box 4
FDA-approved botulinum toxin products

Indication

Cervical dystonia

Axillary hyperhidrosis

Strabismus

Blepharospasm

Urinary incontinence

Migraine headache

Upper limb spasticity

Torticollis

---

have a delay of onset of 1 to 4 days as the toxin is taken up and is able to cleave the SNAP-25 protein. The duration of action is 2 to 4 months, allowing time for the SNAP-25 proteins to regenerate. However, botulinum toxin has other mechanisms of action.

THE ROLE OF BOTULINUM TOXIN IN VASOSPASTIC DISORDERS OF THE HAND

Botulinum toxin has been used to treat vasospasm of digital vessels for more than a decade. The toxin is injected directly into the hand in patients who have primary or secondary Raynaud phenomenon (**Fig. 2**). Botulinum toxin is indicated for patients

Box 5
Off-label uses for botulinum toxin products

Achalasia

Back pain

Carpal tunnel syndrome

Cerebral palsy–related limb spasticity

Chronic anal fissure

Chronic pain

Crow's feet

Delayed gastric emptying

Dystonia

Enlarged prostate

Epilepsy

Epiphora

Essential tremor

Fibromyalgia

Hereditary paraplegia

Interstitial cystitis

Ischemic digits

Lateral epicondylitis

Piriformis syndrome

Pruritus

Raynaud phenomenon

Rhinitis

Sialorrhea

Spasmodic dysphonia

Stuttering

Tardive dyskinesia

Tourette syndrome

Vaginismus

Adapted from Neumeister, Webb KN, Romanelli M. Minimally invasive treatment of Raynaud's phenomenon: the role of botulinum type A. Hand Clinics 2014;30:17–24; with permission.

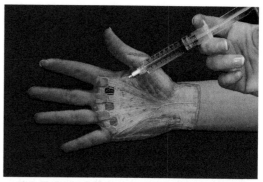

Fig. 2. The reconstituted onabotulinumtoxinA is injected around each neurovascular bundle. Approximately 10 units of onabotulinumtoxinA (2 mL) are used to bathe the neurovascular bundle. (*From* Neumeister MW. Botulinum toxin type a in the treatment of Raynaud's phenomenon. Journ Hand Surg 2010;35(12):2087; with permission.)

who have failed conventional treatment (see **Table 2**). Each drug used for Raynaud vasospasm targets different physiologic sites to induce vasodilation or improve blood flow to the digits. The results of this pharmacologic manipulation vary widely. In the past, patients who did not respond to these medications underwent surgical intervention such as sympathectomies. However, surgery has the potential for complications and has not been uniformly successful; botulinum toxin can now offer these patients an additional option. Multiple case series have shown that, following injection of botulinum toxin, perfusion improves to the digits and the pain associated with the Raynaud resolves almost immediately for most patients, even those patients who have ulcerations.[38–40,60–62]

Observations that injections of botulinum toxin may diminish or even ameliorate chronic pain and improve perfusion in patients with Raynaud have sparked significant basic science research but still the mechanism of action of botulinum toxin is not yet fully elucidated. It seems that botulinum toxin may inhibit the activities of sympathetic and sensory nerves, neurotransmitters, and signal transduction pathways.[57,58,63–65] It is likely that botulinum toxin acts at several sites on vessels and nerves. Vasospasm not only diminishes blood flow but also causes pain. Recurring episodes of the Raynaud phenomenon lead to chronic pain. Chronic pain is propagated by the C-fibers. Injured C-fiber nociceptors become sensitized and undergo significant chemical and biochemical alterations. Adrenergic receptors are upregulated in the sensitized C-fibers. Sympathetic stimulation results in a release of norepinephrine, which acts on the adrenergic receptors to produce both vasoconstriction and pain.[66] Stress and cold each respond to sympathetic discharges and are vasospasm stimuli that result in pain in patients with Raynaud.[64,66,67] The pain may also be the result of stimulation of the release of neurotransmitters such as substance P, which acts as a central nervous system neurotransmitter. Pain nociceptors release substance P and glutamate. Botulinum has been shown to block both substance P and glutamate.

Fonseca and colleagues[6] recently published their hypothesis for the mechanism of action of botulinum toxin, in particular its ability to block vasoconstriction related to cold sensitivity. (**Fig. 3**) The toxin interacts with Rho/Rho kinase to inactivate the Rho kinase. This interaction leads to inhibition of smooth muscle contraction through interference with Ca^{2+} sensitivity and nitric oxide. Laboratory studies on flap viability, vasodilation, and tissue perfusion have shown improvement in tissue perfusion in ischemic models and vessel diameter. In addition, numerous vascular studies in animal models have shown the value of botulinum toxin in inducing vasodilation or preventing thrombosis.[68–73] Improved tissue or flap viability has similarly been documented with the use botulinum toxin.[74–78] Improved tissue viability is presumably through vasodilation and augmented cellular perfusion in these studies.

THE CLINICAL USE OF BOTULINUM TOXIN FOR VASOSPASM

Botulinum toxin holds significant promise for treating vasospasm. The various case series of patients treated with botulinum toxin are listed in **Table 3**.[38–40,59,61] From 75% to 100% of patients report significant improvement of the pain associated with the symptoms of Raynaud phenomenon. Up to 37% of patients have required a repeat injection. Some patients have ongoing relief years after the initial injection. Fregene and colleagues[40] found that 75% of patients experienced a significant reduction in pain, 56% experienced improvement in transcutaneous oxygen saturation, 48% of ulcers healed within 9.5 weeks, and 89% of patients experienced improvements after 1 treatment.

The indications and contraindications for the use of botulinum toxin for vasospastic disorders

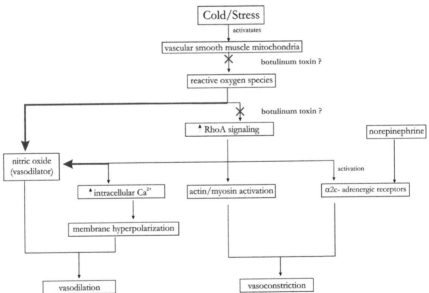

Fig. 3. Pathways involved in vasoconstrictions induced by cold or stress in Raynaud phenomenon. Nitric oxide is a natural vasodilator, and also increases intracellular Ca^{2+}. However, as the skin is exposed to cold in patients with Raynaud phenomenon, the vascular smooth muscle generates reactive oxygen species that are involved in the activation of the RhoA kinase pathway to increase the activity of actin and myosin, leading to vasoconstriction. Furthermore, the activation of the RhoA kinase pathway induces the translocation of α2c adrenergic receptor to the cell surface, where they are stimulated by norepinephrine to create vasoconstriction. Botulinum toxin may block the production of reactive oxygen species, preventing the activation of the RhoA kinase pathway and permitting the unopposed action of nitric oxide leading to vasodilation. Botulinum toxin may alternatively act to increase intracellular Ca^{2+} leading to vasodilation. This pathway is theoretic, based on previous work documented with the RhoA kinase pathway (*red arrows* are inhibitory; *thin black arrows* are stimulatory). (*Adapted from* Fonseca, Abraham D, Ponticos M. Neuronal regulators and vascular dysfunction in Raynaud's phenomenon and systemic sclerosis. Current Vasc Pharm 2009,7(1):36.)

Table 3
Summary of findings from retrospective studies using injected botulinum toxin A to treat patients with Raynaud with ischemic digits

Study	Number of Patients (Male/ Female)	Number of Patients with 1°/2° Raynaud	Average Age in Years (Range)	Percentage with Symptomatic Relief (Number)	Average Length of Follow-up in Months (Maximum)	Average Duration of Pain Relief in Months (Range)	Number of Complications (%)
Sycha et al,[62] 2004	2 (0/2)	1/1	50.5 (19–63)	100 (2/2)	1.75 (2)	1.75 (1.5–2)	None
Van Beeket al,[39] 2007	11 (2/9)	1/10	50.8 (23–70)	100 (11/11)	9.6 (30)	Not reported	Temporary intrinsic muscle weakness, 3 (27)
Fregene et al,[40] 2009	26 (12/14)	15/11	55 (37–72)	75 (19/6)	18 (45)	Not Reported	Temporary intrinsic muscle weakness, 6 (23) Transient dysesthesia, injected distal, 1 (4)
Neumeister et al,[38] 2009	19 (7/12)	13/6	44.1 (15–72)	84 (16/19)	Not reported (59)	23.4 (0.5–59)	Temporary intrinsic muscle weakness, 3 (16)
Neumeister,[60] 2010	33 (14/19)	23/10	43.0 (15–72)	84 (28/33)	(103)	(0.5–103)	Temporary intrinsic muscle weakness, 7 (21%)

Adapted from Neumeister, Webb KN, Romanelli M. Minimally invasive treatment of Raynaud's phenomenon: the role of botulinum type A. Hand Clinics 2014;30:22; with permission.

Box 6
Indications for botulinum toxin in patients with ischemic digits

- Raynaud phenomenon
- Vascular insufficiency not amenable to bypass surgery

Adapted from Neumeister MW, Webb KN, Romanelli M. Minimally invasive treatment of Raynaud phenomenon – the role of botulinum type A. Hand Clinics 2014;30;1:17–24; with permission.

Box 7
The contraindications for the use of botulinum toxin A

- Known allergies
- Pregnancy
- Breast-feeding mothers
- Active infections
- Myasthenia gravis
- Patients on medications that decrease neuromuscular transmission:
  - Calcium channel blockers
  - Penicillamine
  - Aminoglycosides
  - Lincosamides
  - Polymyxins
  - Magnesium sulfate
  - Anticholinesterases
  - Succinylcholine
  - Quinidine

Adapted from Neumeister MW, Webb KN, Romanelli M. Minimally invasive treatment of Raynaud phenomenon – the role of botulinum type A. Hand Clinics 2014;30;1:17–24; with permission.

are listed in **Boxes 6** and **7** respectively. Clinical examples are included to show the efficiency of botulinum (**Figs. 4–8**) There are still several questions to be answered with the use of botulinum toxin in vasospastic disorders. The exact dose response curve has not been elucidated, meaning that lower doses might suffice. In contrast, perhaps greater doses are required for those patients who did not respond as well as expected. Understanding the mechanism of action of botulinum toxin is important because it may help clinicians to define which patients are going to respond better than others to the toxin injections.

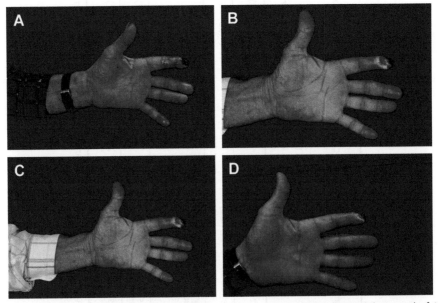

Fig. 4. A patient with recalcitrant Raynaud and an ischemic ulcer on the index finger (*A*). A total of 100 units of onabotulinumtoxinA were injected into the hand. Immediate relief of pain was reported and the perfusion improved. The ulcers healed except for an area of exposed distal phalanx that required a revision amputation (*B–D*). The patient remains symptom free at 6-year follow-up.

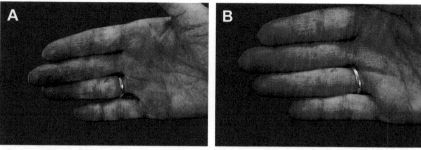

Fig. 5. Patient with Raynaud who underwent onabotulinumtoxinA injections (*A*). There is observable improvement in perfusion after the injections (*B*).

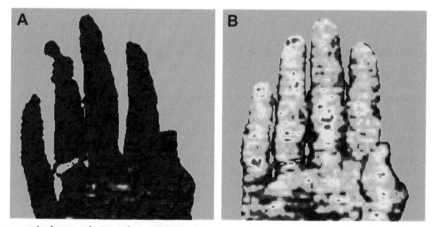

Fig. 6. Laser scans before perfusion of a patient with Raynaud injected with 100 units of botulinum toxin type A (*A*). A marked increase in perfusion was observed after the injection (*B*).

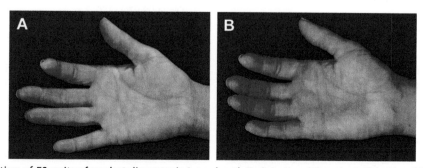

Fig. 7. Injection of 50 units of onabotulinumtoxinA per hand. Preinjection (*A*) and postinjection (*B*).

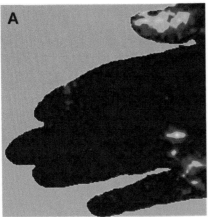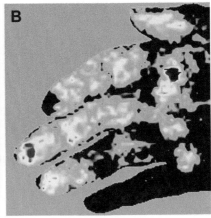

Fig. 8. Before (*A*) and after (*B*) botulinum toxin laser scans of a patient who had previous amputations as a result of severe digital ischemia and necrosis. The patient had previous digital sympathectomies that did not improve the perfusion of the digits. The remaining digits had become ischemic and the patient underwent onabotulinumtoxinA injections to improve perfusion. The remaining digits were salvaged.

It may be that some patients have an immunologic resistance to botulinum toxin; Borodic[79] observed decreasing effectiveness of botulinum injections after repeated treatment of facial rhytids. Earlier, Greene and colleagues[80] described resistance to botulinum toxin after repeated injections for patients with torticollis. It is conceivable that some patients have localized resistance to the toxin despite never having previous injections of the toxin. However, it is more likely that the patients with vasospastic disorders who do not respond as well as others may have alterations in the mechanisms described earlier.

SUMMARY

At present, botulinum injections offer a low-risk method for the treatment of symptomatic Raynaud phenomenon. Although the mechanism has not been fully elucidated, this finding provides patients with another option for medical management before moving to sympathectomy. Repeated injections may be required.

ACKNOWLEDGMENTS

The author acknowledges the dedication of Evyn Neumeister, BA, for her hours of work helping to write and prepare this article.

REFERENCES

1. Bakst R, Merola JF, Franks AG, et al. Raynaud's phenomenon: pathogenesis and management. J Am Acad Dermatol 2008;59(4):633–53.
2. de Trafford JC, Lafferty K, Potter CE, et al. An epidemiological survey of Raynaud's phenomenon. Eur J Vasc Surg 1988;2:167–70.
3. Department of Health and Human Services, Public Health Service, National Institutes of Health, et al. Questions and answers about Raynaud's phenomenon. NIH; 2001. Publication No. 06–4911, Revised June 2006. Available at: http://vickiehonea.com/raynaudsRP_04.pdf.
4. Garcia-Carrasco M, Jimenez-Hernandez M, Escarcega RO, et al. Treatment of Raynaud's phenomenon. Autoimmun Rev 2008;8:62–8.
5. Bowling JC, Dowd PM. Raynaud's disease. Lancet 2003;361:2078–80.
6. Fonseca C, Abraham D, Ponticos M. Neuronal regulators and vascular dysfunction in Raynaud's phenomenon and systemic sclerosis. Curr Vasc Pharmacol 2009;7(1):34–9.
7. Ramien M, Brassard A. The challenge of scleroderma ulcers. J Cutan Med Surg 2009;13(Suppl 1):S42–8.
8. Nihtgyanova SI, Brough GM, Black CM, et al. Clinical burden of digital vasculopathy in limited and diffuse cutaneous systemic sclerosis. Ann Rheum Dis 2008;67(1):120–3.
9. Morris JL, Jobling P, Gibbins IL. Differential inhibition by botulinum neurotoxin A of cotransmitters released from autonomic vasodilator neurons. Am J Physiol Heart Circ Physiol 2001;28:H2124–32.
10. Silveri F, De Angelis R, Poggi A, et al. Relative roles of endothelial cell damage and platelet activation in primary Raynaud's phenomenon (RP) and RP secondary to systemic sclerosis. Scand J Rheumatol 2001;30:290–6.
11. Rosato E, Letizia C, Proietti M, et al. Plasma adrenomedullin and endothelin-1 levels are reduced and

Raynaud's phenomenon improved by daily tadalafil administration in male patients with systemic sclerosis. J Biol Regul Homeost Agents 2009;23:23–9.

12. Durham PL, Cady R, Cady R. Regulation of calcitonin gene-related peptide secretion from trigeminal nerve cells by botulinum toxin type A: implications for migraine therapy. Headache 2004 Jan;44(1): 35–42 [discussion: 42–3].

13. Edwards CM, Marshall JM, Pugh M. Cardiovascular responses evoked mild cool stimuli in primary Raynaud's disease: the role of endothelin. Clin Sci 1999;96:577.

14. Freedman RR, Girgis R, Mayes M. Endothelial and adrenergic dysfunction in Raynaud's phenomenon and scleroderma. J Rheumatol 1999;26(11):2386–8.

15. Lazzerini PE, Capecchi PL, Bisogno S, et al. Homocysteine and Raynaud's phenomenon: a review. Autoimmun Rev 2010;9:181–7.

16. Leppert J, Ringqvis A, Ahlner J. Seasonal variations in cyclic GMP response on whole-body cooling in women with primary Raynaud's phenomenon. Clin Sci 1997;93:175.

17. McMahon HT, Foran P, Dolly JO, et al. Tetanus toxin and botulinum toxins type A and B inhibit glutamate, gamma-aminobutyric acid, aspartate, and met-enkephalin release from synaptosomes. Clues to the locus of action. J Biol Chem 1992;267(30): 21338–43.

18. Muller-Ladner U, Distler O, Ibba-Manneschi L, et al. Mechanisms of vascular damage in systemic sclerosis. Autoimmunity Oct 2009;42(7):587–95.

19. Duprez DA. Role of the renin-angiotensin-aldosterone system in vascular remodeling and inflammation: a clinical review. J Hypertens 2006; 24:983–91.

20. Kawaguchi Y, Takagi K, Hara M, et al. Angiotensin II in the lesional skin of systemic sclerosis patients contributes to tissue fibrosis via angiotensin II type 1 receptors. Arthritis Rheumatol 2004;50:216–26.

21. Sgonc R, Gruschwitz MS, Boeck G, et al. Endothelial cell apoptosis in systemic sclerosis is induced by antibody-dependent cell-mediated cytotoxicity via CD95. Arthritis Rheum 2000;43:2550–62.

22. Flavahan NA, Vanhoutte PM. Endothelial cell signaling and endothelial dysfunction. Am J Hypertens 1995;8(Suppl):28S–41S.

23. Droste H, Wollersheim H, Reyenga J, et al. Vascular and humoral sympathetic nervous system reactively during mental arithmatic in primary Raynaud's phenomenon. Int Angiol 1990;9:84–9.

24. Bunker CB, Goldsmith PC, Leslie TA, et al. Calcitonin gene-related peptide, endothelin-1, the cutaneous microvasculature and Raynaud's phenomenon. Br J Dermatol 1996;134:399–406.

25. Bunker CB, Terenghi G, Springall DR, et al. Deficiency of calcitonin gene-related peptide in Raynaud's phenomenon. Lancet 1990;336:1530–3.

26. Bunker CB, Reavlety C, O'Shaughnessy DJ, et al. Calcitonin gene-related peptide in treatment of severe peripheral vascular insufficiency in Raynaud's phenomenon. Lancet 1993;342:80–3.

27. Generini S, Seibold JR, Matucci-Cerinic M. Estrogens and neuropeptides in Raynaud's phenomenon. Rheum Dis Clin North Am 2005;31:177–86.

28. Chotani MA, Flavahan S, Mitra S, et al. Silent alpha (2C)-adrenergic receptors enable cold-induced vasoconstriction in cutaneous arteries. Am J Physiol Heart Circ Physiol 2000;278:H1075–83.

29. Bailey SR, Eid AH, Mitra S, et al. Rho kinase mediates cold-induced construction of cutaneous arteries: role of alpha2C-adrenoceptor translocation. Circ Res 2004;94:1367–74.

30. Bailey SR, Mitra S, Flavahan S, et al. Reactive oxygen species from smooth muscle mitochondria initiate cold-induced constriction of cutaneous arteries. Am J Physiol Heart Circ Physiol 2005;289: H243–50.

31. Furspan PB, Chatterjee S, Freedman RR. Increased tyrosine phosphorylation mediates the cooling-induced contraction and increase vascular reactivity of Raynaud's disease. Arthritis Rheum 2004;50: 1578–85.

32. Furspan PB, Chatterjee S, Mayes MD, et al. Cooling-induced contraction and protein tyrosine kinase activity of isolated arterioles in secondary Raynaud's phenomenon. Rheumatology 2005;44:488–94.

33. Lau CS, McLaren M, Saniabadi A, et al. Increased whole blood platelet aggregation in patients with Raynaud's phenomenon with or without systemic sclerosis. Scand J Rheumatol 1993;22:97–101.

34. LeRoy EC. Systemic sclerosis: a vascular perspective. Rheum Dis Clin North Am 1996;22:675–94.

35. Flavahan NA, Flavahan S, Mitra S, et al. The vasculopathy of Raynaud's phenomenon and scleroderma. Rheum Dis Clin North Am 2003;29:275–91.

36. Henness S, Wigley FM. Current drug therapy for scleroderma and secondary Raynaud's phenomenon: evidence-based review. Curr Opin Rheumatol 2007;19(6):611–8.

37. Lambova SN, Muller-Ladner U. New lines in therapy of Raynaud's phenomenon. Rheumatol Int 2009;29: 355–63.

38. Neumeister MW, Chambers CB, Herron MS, et al. Botox therapy for ischemic digits. Plast Reconstr Surg 2009;124(1):191–201.

39. Van Beek AL, Lim PK, Gear AJL, et al. Management of vasospastic disorders with botulinum toxin A. Plast Reconstr Surg 2007;119:217.

40. Fregene A, Ditmars D, Siddiqui A. Botulinum toxin type A: a treatment option for digital ischemia in patients with Raynaud's phenomenon. J Hand Surg Am 2009;34(3):446–52.

41. Koman LA, Smith BP, Smith TL. Vascular disorders. In: Green DP, Hotchkiss RN, Pederson WC, editors.

Greens operative hand surgery. New York: Churchill Livingstone; 1999. p. 2254–302.

42. Baumhaekel M, Scheffler P, Boehm M. Use of tadalafil in a patient with a secondary Raynaud's phenomenon not responding to sildenafil. Microvasc Res 2005;69(3):178–9.

43. Baak SW. Treatment of Raynaud's phenomena with PDE-5 inhibitors, Cialis (tadalafil) in patients with scleroderma and lupus. Arthritis Rheum 2005; 52(Suppl 9):S169.

44. Cheung GT, Lau CS, Kumana CR. Phosphodiesterase 5-inhibitors relieve symptoms of severe Raynaud's phenomenon. Ann Rheum Dis 2004; 64(Suppl 2):211.

45. Colglazier CL, Sutej PG, O'Rourke KS. Severe refractory fingertip ulcerations in a patient with scleroderma: successful treatment with sildenafil. J Rheumatol 2005;32(12):2440–2.

46. Caglayan E, Huntgeburth M, Karasch T, et al. Phosphodiesterase type 5 inhibition is a novel therapeutic option in Raynaud's disease. Arch Intern Med 2006; 166:231–3.

47. Carlino G. Treatment of Raynaud's phenomenon with tadalafil, a phosphodiesterase-5 inhibitor. Ann Rheum Dis 2005;64(Suppl 3):258.

48. Sandorfi N, Jimenez SA. Treatment of digital ulceration due to Raynaud's phenomenon (RP) with long acting phosphodiesterase 5 (PDE5) inhibitors: tadalafil. Ann Rheum Dis 2007;66(Suppl 2):223.

49. Kumar N, Griffiths B, Allen J. Thermographic and symptomatic effects of a single dose of sildenafil citrate on Raynaud's phenomenon in patients with systemic sclerosis: a potential treatment. J Rheumatol 2006;33(9):1918–9.

50. Kamata Y, Kamimura T, Iwamoto M, et al. Comparable effects of sildenafil citrate and alprostadil on severe Raynaud's phenomenon in a patient with systemic sclerosis. Clin Exp Dermatol 2005;30: 435–56.

51. Lin CS, Lin G, Xin ZC, et al. Expression, distribution, and regulation of phosphodiesterase 5. Curr Pharm Des 2006;12:3439–57.

52. Pakozdi A, Howell K, Black CM, et al. Addition of the short term phosphodiesterase-5 inhibitor sildenafil to iloprost therapy for scleroderma digital vasculopathy. Arthritis Rheum 2007;56(Suppl):825.

53. Schiopu E, Hsu VM, Impens AJ, et al. Controlled trial of tadalafil in Raynaud's phenomenon (RP) secondary to systemic sclerosis. Arthritis Rheum 2006; 54(Suppl 2):505.

54. Zamiri B, Koman AL, Smith BP, et al. Double-blind, placebo-controlled trail of sildenafil for the management of primary Raynaud's phenomenon. Ann Rheum Dis 2004;63(Suppl3):342.

55. Snipe PT, Sommer H. Studies on Botulinus toxin: 3. Acid precipitation of Botulinus toxin. J Infect Dis 1928;43(2):152–60.

56. Burgen AS, Dickens F, Zatman LJ. The action of botulinum toxin on the neuromuscular junction. J Physiol 1949;109(1–2):10–24.

57. Setler P. Therapeutic use of botulinum toxins: background and history. Clin J Pain 2002;18(6):S119–24.

58. Cheng CM, Chen JS, Patel RP. Unlabled uses of botulinum toxins: a review, part 1. Am J Health Syst Pharm 2006;63(2):145–52.

59. Aoki KR. Pharmacology and immunology of botulinum toxin serotypes. J Neurol 2001;248(Suppl 1):3–10.

60. Neumeister MW. Botulinum toxin type A in the treatment of Raynaud's phenomenon. J Hand Surg 2010; 35A:2085–92.

61. Neumeister MW, Webb KN, Romanelli M. Minimally invasive treatment of Raynaud's phenomenon: the role of botulinum type A. Hand Clin 2014;30:17–34.

62. Sycha T, Graninger M, Auff E, et al. Botulinum toxin in the treatment of Raynaud's phenomenon: a pilot study. Eur J Clin Invest 2004;34:312–3.

63. Cui M, Khanijou S, Rubino J, et al. Subcutaneous administration of botulinum toxin A reduces formalin-induced pain. Pain 2004;107:125–33.

64. Devor M, Wall PD. Cross-excitation in dorsal root ganglia of nerve-injured and intact rats. J Neurophysiol 1990;64(6):1733–46.

65. Halperin JL, Cohen RA, Coffman JD. Digital vasodilatation during mental stress in patients with Raynaud's disease. Cardiovasc Res 1983;17:671–7.

66. Colhado OC, Boeing M, Ortega LB. Botulinum toxin in pain treatment. Rev Bras Anestesiol 2009;59(3): 366–81.

67. Martinez RM, Saponaro A, Dragagna G, et al. Cutaneous circulation in Raynaud's phenomenon during emotional stress: a morphological and functional study using capillaroscopy and laser-Doppler. Int Angiol 1992;11:316–20.

68. Fathi M, Fathi H, Mazloumi M, et al. Preventive effect of botulinum toxin A in microanastomotic thrombosis: a rabbit model. J Plast Reconstr Aesthet Surg 2010;63(10):e720–4.

69. Janz BA, Thomas PR, Fanua SP, et al. Prevention of anastomotic thrombosis by botulinum toxin B after acute injury in a rat model. J Hand Surg Am 2011; 36(1):1585–91.

70. Park BY, Kim HK, Kim WS, et al. The effect of botulinum toxin B pretreatment to the blood flow in the microvascular anastomosis. Ann Plast Surg 2014; 72(2):214–9.

71. Murakami E, Iwata H, Imaizumi M, et al. Prevention of arterial graft spasm by botulinum toxin: an invitro experiment. Interact Cardiovasc Thorac Surg 2009;9(3):395–8.

72. Clemens MW, Higgins JP, Wilgis EF. Prevention of anastomotic thrombosis by botulinum toxin-A in an animal model. Plast Reconstr Surg 2009;123(1): 64–70.

73. Upton J, Garcia J, Liao E. Botox to the rescue. Plast Reconstr Surg 2009;123(1):38e.
74. Kim YS, Roh TS, Lee WJ, et al. The effect of botulinum toxin A on skin flap survival in rats. Wound Repair Regen 2009;17(3):411–7.
75. Arnold PB, Merritt W, Rodeheaver GT, et al. Effects of perivascular botulinum toxin-A application on vascular smooth muscle and flap viability in the rat. Ann Plast Surg 2009;62(5):463–7.
76. Arnold PB, Fang T, Songcharoen SJ, et al. Inflammatory response and survival of pedicled abdominal flaps in a rat model after perivascular application of botulinum toxin type A. Plast Reconstr Surg 2014;133(4):491e–8e.

77. Schweizer DF, Schweizer R, Zhang S, et al. Botulinum toxin A and B raise blood flow and increase survival of critically ischemic skin flaps. J Surg Res 2013;184:1205–13.
78. Stone AV, Koman LA, Callahan MF, et al. The effect of botulinum neurotoxin A on blood flow in rats: a potential mechanism for the treatment of Raynaud's phenomenon. J Hand Surg 2012;37(4):795–802.
79. Borodic G. Immunologic resistance after repeated botulinum toxin A injections for facial rhytids. Ophthal Plast Reconstr Surg 2006;6(22):239.
80. Greene P, Fahn S, Diamond B. Development of resistance to botulinum toxin type A in patients with torticollis. Mov Disord 1994;9:213.

Vasospastic Disorders of the Hand

Vascular Injuries in the Upper Extremity in Athletes

Tristan de Mooij, MD, Audra A. Duncan, MD,
Sanjeev Kakar, MD, MRCS, MBA*

KEYWORDS

- Vascular injury • Athlete • Upper extremity • Thoracic outlet syndrome
- Quadrilateral space syndrome • Posterior humeral circumflex injuries
- Hypothenar hammer syndrome • Digital ischemia

KEY POINTS

- Overhead motions may impinge on neurovascular bundles at the shoulder region through compression; for example, by the humeral head, muscle inflammation, or cysts.
- Athletes may benefit from instrument modification, motion analysis and adjustment, as well as equipment enhancement to limit exposure to blunt trauma or impingement.
- Arterial aneurysms caused by repetitive compression may require surgical treatment with ligation or revascularization to prevent or treat limb-threatening distal embolization.

INTRODUCTION

Upper extremity arterial injuries can occur in athletes performing repetitive, high-stress, or high-impact arm motions. In elite throwers, the internal rotation velocity of the arm during the acceleration phase reaches more than 7000° per second.[1] The increased functional range of shoulder girdle motion, which these athletes require for competition, causes increased stresses on the vascular structures within the shoulder and upper extremity.[2] In addition, muscle hypertrophy and fatigue-induced joint translation may incite impingement on critical neurovasculature.[2] The initial presentation of these injuries often mimics more common musculoskeletal injuries found in these athletes, and therefore a thorough evaluation is essential to establish the diagnosis in a timely fashion.[3] Arterial disease usually presents with muscular pain at the extremes of effort, acute ischemia from thrombosis or embolus, or an artery may be ruptured during certain sporting activities.[4]

Symptoms of hand ischemia may occur in the form of Raynaud syndrome or large or small arterial occlusion. Athletes particularly at risk include baseball and softball players, but injuries have been reported in volleyball players, weight lifters, swimmers, and many others.[5,6] Clinical diagnoses are often confirmed with noninvasive vascular laboratory testing and contrast imaging. Most cases can be successfully treated conservatively by means of avoidance of the causative factor as well as instrument and/or equipment modification. However, patients with arterial or venous occlusions and/or aneurysm formation requiring surgical management may have excellent functional outcomes allowing return to play.

This article discusses upper extremity vascular disorders in athletes caused by embolic syndromes (quadrilateral space syndrome, humeral head compression of the axillary artery, and arterial thoracic outlet syndrome [TOS]), vein compression (venous TOS), and direct digital

Disclosure: The authors have nothing to disclose of relevance to this article.
Mayo Clinic, 200 1st Street South West, Rochester, MN 55905, USA
* Corresponding author.
E-mail address: kakar.sanjeev@mayo.edu

artery injury (hypothenar hammer syndrome), and evaluates pathophysiology, diagnosis, and treatment.

QUADRILATERAL SPACE SYNDROME

The posterior circumflex humeral artery (PCHA) arises from the distal third of the axillary artery and, together with the axillary nerve, courses through the quadrilateral space, which is bordered by the teres minor superiorly, the teres major inferiorly, the humeral shaft laterally, and the long head of the triceps medially. Reported initially in 1983 by Cahill and Palmer,[7] 18 patients were identified with point tenderness over the quadrilateral space posteriorly that was aggravated by forward flexion and/or abduction and external rotation of the humerus (the cocked position). Included in the differential diagnosis of quadrilateral space syndrome is suprascapular neuropathy, which is frequently seen in volleyball players (ie, so-called volleyball shoulder). However, suprascapular neuropathy is thought to be a mononeuropathy without vascular compromise.[8] Angiographic confirmation of the quadrilateral space syndrome may be shown with occlusion of the posterior humeral circumflex artery with the arm in abduction and external rotation. Chronic compression and repeated trauma over the artery can occur in overhand motion athletes such as baseball pitchers and volleyball players and may result in artery occlusion or

aneurysm formation causing subsequent embolization (**Fig. 1**).[9] In addition, inflammation of any or all of the muscular borders of the quadrilateral space may constrict the space around the PCHA and axillary nerve and cause gradual onset of symptoms.[8] Other hypotheses regarding the potential mechanisms of quadrilateral space syndrome include (1) traction by the pectoralis major muscle on the PCHA,[10] (2) fixation of the PCHA to the proximal humerus caused by its circumflex course making it prone to traction and subsequent intima injury (this hypothesis is supported by the report from Durham and colleagues[11] identifying positional axillary arterial compression with concomitant PCHA occlusion), (3) glenohumeral instability or glenoid labral cyst compressing the PCHA, and (4) chronic overuse with subsequent fibrous bands causing compression within the quadrilateral space.[12]

As with many intermittent compressive syndromes of the upper extremity, in the absence of fixed compression or aneurysm, initial treatment should include correction of the underlying insult (such as poor biomechanics). Physical therapy should focus on gradually rehabilitating the shoulder girdle to prevent repeated compression. If this fails, or aneurysm is present, surgical treatment may be necessary with decompression of the quadrilateral space.[7,13] In the series by Cahill and Palmer,[7] surgical decompression in 18 patients resulted in cure in 8, improvement in 8, and no improvement in 2. If an aneurysm has developed,

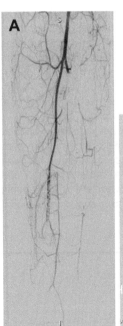

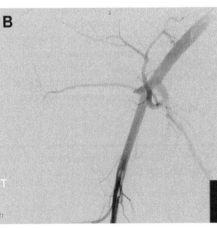

Fig. 1. Digital contrast angiogram of a 20-year-old female volleyball player with acute onset of right upper extremity digital ischemia. (*A*) Abrupt occlusion of the radial artery 1 cm from its origin and extensive thromboembolism of distal third of the ulnar artery. (*B*) Proximal imaging identified abrupt occlusion of the PCHA, which was subsequently identified as aneurysmal.

treatment is ligation of the posterior humeral circumflex artery, as long as the anterior humeral circumflex artery is preserved to prevent avascular necrosis.[14]

HUMERAL HEAD COMPRESSION OF THE AXILLARY ARTERY

Similar to quadrilateral space syndrome, humeral head compression of the axillary artery also occurs with overhead motions or with striking motions when the arm is abducted and externally rotated. During those motions, the humeral head can be displaced downward, pushing it against the axillary artery.[15,16] Patients are typically athletes in overhead motion sports, and often present with arm fatigue, decreased ability to pitch, numbness and coolness in the fingers, and distal embolization. Diagnosis can be made by ultrasonography evaluation before and after overhead maneuvers showing decreased flow through the axillary artery with stress.[17]

As with quadrilateral space syndrome, without fixed arterial injury initial treatment is modification of upper extremity ergonomics, such as a change in pitching motion. If symptoms do not improve or there is arterial injury, saphenous vein patch or bypass may be indicated.[11,18] Rehabilitation after operation is usually successful at allowing patients to return to competitive sports.[11,19]

VASCULAR THORACIC OUTLET

In contrast with the compressive syndromes discussed earlier, TOS can affect both arteries and veins. Axillosubclavian vascular injury may occur in young, healthy individuals who present with sudden arm swelling, cyanosis, or emboli following vigorous activity, and is caused by compression of the axillary or subclavian vein or artery at the junction of the first rib and clavicle (**Fig. 2**).[20] Although most patients with TOS (95%) present with neurologic symptoms, a small percentage (3%) may have venous compression, and 2% may have arterial compromise.[21] Arterial lesions may occur in the setting of a congenital cervical rib or anomalous first rib. Venous effort thrombosis (VET) is a potential cause of disability in young, active patients and often occurs in young athletes, interfering greatly with their lifestyles.[22,23]

The borders of the thoracic outlet, including the anterior and middle scalene muscles, first rib, or cervical rib, may cause intermittent compression of the axillary or subclavian artery. Over time, with repetitive motion, the artery may become aneurysmal with intraluminal thrombus and subsequent emboli or develop intimal hyperplasia. Patients may present with effort fatigue, the sensation of coolness, and a reduction in arm blood pressure with positional maneuvers. In 1986, Fields and colleagues[24] published a case report of a catastrophic stroke in a major league pitcher secondary to subclavian artery in situ thrombosis with proximal thrombus propagation. Men may be slightly more affected than women.[11] On physical examination, a loss of radial pulse with extended arm stress test maneuvers is typically found, but that finding has a low specificity. Cervical ribs, if large, can be palpated in the neck in thin patients. Tenderness over the anterior scalene muscle is often noted. In the setting of emboli from subclavian aneurysms, petechiae or livedo reticularis may be seen in the affected hand.

Initial imaging studies should include C-spine or chest roentgenogram to rule out cervical rib (**Fig. 3**), and ultrasonography with abduction to assess compression of the axillary and subclavian arteries. Ultrasonography may be limited by body habitus, especially if the affected segment of artery is directly under the clavicle. Contrast imaging, either with conventional angiography or computed tomography angiography, done in resting

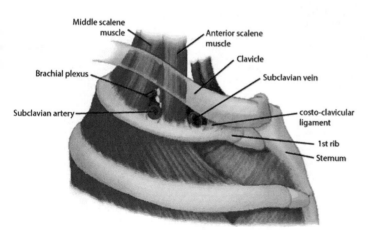

Middle scalene muscle
Anterior scalene muscle
Clavicle
Brachial plexus
Subclavian vein
Subclavian artery
costo-clavicular ligament
1st rib
Sternum

Fig. 2. Normal anatomy of the thoracic outlet. (*From* Urschel HC, Patel AN. Surgery remains the most effective treatment for Paget-Schroetter syndrome: 50 years' experience. Ann Thorac Surg 2008;86:255; with permission.)

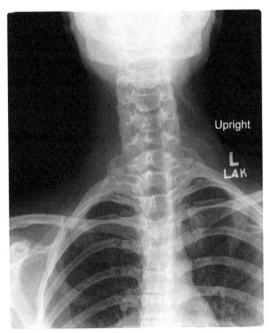

Fig. 3. Upright cervical radiograph of 22-year-old softball player with right arterial TOS shows a large cervical rib.

and abducted positions, provides valuable information about the arteries, including an assessment of aneurysm if present (**Fig. 4**).[25]

If an arterial aneurysm is present, operative treatment is required to prevent potentially debilitation emboli to the hand. If emboli are already present, thrombolysis may be effective to treated distal, painful lesions, if done in a timely manner.[26]

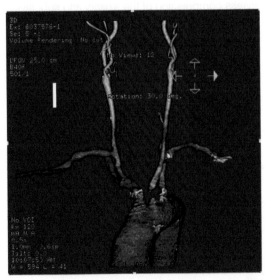

Fig. 4. Computed tomography of an 18-year-old basketball player with arterial TOS identified bilateral subclavian artery aneurysms.

Surgical treatment of subclavian aneurysms includes supraclavicular or infraclavicular artery exposure, decompression of the thoracic outlet with first and cervical rib resection, scalenectomy, and artery replacement with saphenous vein or prosthetic depending on the artery size.[26] Patients can often return to full sports activity and often do not require long-term anticoagulation in the absence of a hypercoagulable state.

VENOUS COMPRESSION

Axillosubclavian venous thrombosis may occur in young, healthy individuals who present with sudden arm swelling and cyanosis following vigorous activity, and is caused by compression of the subclavian vein at the junction of the first rib and clavicle.[20] This type of TOS is more commonly known as VET or Paget-Schroetter syndrome.[27–29] Although most patients with TOS (95%) present with neurologic symptoms, a small percentage (2%–3%) may have VET.[21] At present, there is no consensus regarding the optimal management of VET with regard to acute subclavian vein thrombosis, timing of surgery, surgical approach, and the need for anticoagulation following surgical decompression of the thoracic outlet. However, in athletes, prompt treatment with thrombolytics if indicated followed by prompt TOS decompression is typically favored to shorten the period of inactivity and reduce time required for anticoagulation.

Patients with VET often present with a sudden onset of arm swelling. In some cases this has been preceded by episodes of arm swelling with activity that was self-limited. As with sudden onset of lower extremity swelling, the venous outflow should be investigated promptly by duplex ultrasonography to confirm or rule out the presence of a deep venous thrombosis (**Fig. 5**). In Urschel and Patel's[20] series of 626 patients, all had venous distension, 618 had subcutaneous venous collaterals around the shoulder, 602 had arm swelling,

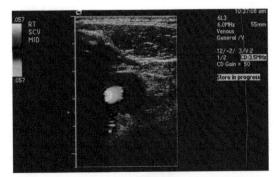

Fig. 5. Duplex ultrasonography of a 16-year-old weight lifter with a right subclavian deep vein thrombosis.

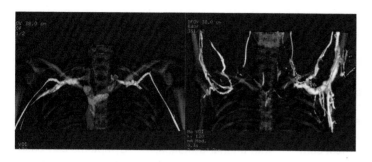

Fig. 6. Computed tomography venogram of a 16-year-old softball player with significant arm swelling after pitching shows occlusion of both subclavian veins with abduction and external rotation.

591 had bluish discoloration, 207 had aching pain with exercise, 62 had cervical ribs, and 24 had minimal symptoms. Diagnosis is often obtained with a combination of history and physical examination. If the patient has minimal symptoms, but TOS compression signs (such as Adson maneuver or hyperabduction) are positive, duplex ultrasonography and a cervical spine radiograph to rule out a cervical rib should be done. If the duplex examination is equivocal or unavailable, venogram either with conventional imaging, computed tomography venography, or magnetic resonance venography (MRV) is performed (**Fig. 6**).

As with arterial TOS, surgical treatment often requires TOS decompression combined with vein reconstruction as indicated. If the vein is severely disease, venoplasty with saphenous vein or bovine pericardium patch or interposition vein bypass may be necessary. If venous reconstruction is required, patients should receive long-term anticoagulation.

HYPOTHENAR HAMMER SYNDROME

Hypothenar hammer syndrome (HHS) is an overuse syndrome to the hand caused by vascular disorder of the ulnar artery or the superficial palmar arch.[30,31] Originally described by Von Rosen[32] in the 1930s, Conn and colleagues[31] described its pathophysiology and coined the term HHS. Although previously thought to be uncommon, HHS is now understood to be particularly highly prevalent in athletes and manual laborers.

Anatomy of the Ulnar Artery and the Pathophysiology of Hypothenar Hammer Syndrome

The radial and ulnar arteries provide the main blood supply to the wrist and hand, and anastomose at several levels forming vascular arches. Within the Guyon canal, the ulnar artery bifurcates at the level of the hamate into the deep and superficial palmar branches. Guyon canal's is divided into 3 zones: zone 1 is proximal to the division of the ulnar nerve, zone 2 contains the deep motor branch, and zone 3 contains the superficial branch of the ulnar nerve.[33] The superficial palmar branch of the ulnar artery crosses the hypothenar muscles for 2 cm before penetrating the palmar aponeurosis and forming its terminal arch (**Fig. 7**).[34,35] This segment is highly susceptible to blunt trauma

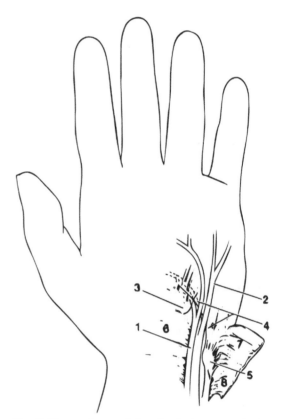

Fig. 7. The anatomy of the distal ulnar tunnel. The relationship of the ulnar artery in the Guyon canal is depicted along with anatomic landmarks. 1, ulnar artery; 2, superficial branch of the ulnar nerve; 3, hamulus; 4, fibrous arch of the hypothenar muscles; 5, pisiform; 6, transverse carpal ligament; 7, palmaris brevis; 8, palmar carpal ligament. (*From* Gross MS, Gelberman RH. The anatomy of the distal ulnar tunnel. Clin Orthop Relat Res 1985;(196):238–47; with permission.)

given its relative superficial location. In addition, because of its tethering to the deep palmar branch, the artery is immobile and as a result can easily be compressed against the adjacent hook of hamate.[34] These predisposing factors can lead to aneurysmal degeneration via increasing vascular wall weakness, a process that is further accelerated by mechanical stress generated by the ensuing altered hemodynamics.[36] These mechanisms make the ulnar artery the most common site for true and false aneurysms of the upper extremity, and explain the epidemiologic age differences between athlete and nonathlete populations based on age and intensity of exposure.[36]

Aneurysmal degeneration may have both congenital and acquired components. Some patients may be predisposed because of intrinsically abnormal bilateral ulnar arteries with a typical corkscrew appearance, reminiscent of fibromuscular dysplasia.[37] Others may be predisposed because of a more proximal course of the artery to the hook of the hamate.[38] Anatomic studies have found variable relationships between the ulnar artery and the hamulus, with the average distance of the artery to the hamulus ranging from 2.8 to 7 mm ulnar to 2 to 7.8 mm radially.[39,40]

Epidemiology

Although initially recognized as a potential occupational hazard among manual laborers, craftsmen, and habitual hand hammerers, this disorder can be prevalent among athletes.[41,42] Athletes exposed to regular blunt trauma to the hypothenar eminence are submitted to exposure mechanisms that are similar to those experienced by manual laborers. However, this predisposition may be further accentuated by modifications to athletes' instruments, poor protective gear, and the intensity of their training.[2,43] Case reports have been published from a wide variety of sports, including baseball, softball,[18,44,45] basketball,[46] volleyball,[47] cricket, football,[48] golf,[49] badminton,[49,50] frisbee,[18] breakdancing,[51] karate,[31] squash, soccer (goalkeepers),[52] hockey,[41,53] handball,[48] ice hockey,[43] tennis,[54,55] cycling,[56,57] snowboarding,[58] and weight lifting (**Table 1**).[59] This variety indicates that a larger patient population may be at risk, and recognition of the condition is important to avoid poor outcomes.[42,60]

Clinical Presentation

The clinical presentation of HHS depends on anatomic variations, the severity of the vascular disorder, and the development of collateral blood flow. In more than 90% of patients, the dominant hand is affected.[61] Because the long finger is the last digit to be vascularized by the superficial palmar arch, this digit is most prone to ischemia.[37] Patients may present with acute paleness and numbness in the hand, ulceration, necrosis, or chronic symptoms such as Raynaud phenomenon or cramping with activity, as well as ulnar nerve compression symptoms. In addition, pulsations and a thrill or bruit may be appreciated. Young athletes often present with occlusions and less often with arterial dilatation.[41–43] Symptoms can occur gradually or acutely, but usually present unilaterally, in contrast with most systemic diseases.

Differential Diagnosis

HHS has a broad differential diagnosis including Raynaud disease, Raynaud phenomenon, scleroderma, systemic lupus erythematosus, thromboangiitis obliterans (Buerger disease), arterial embolus of cardiac origin, atherosclerosis with secondary thrombosis, TOS, and hand-arm vibration syndrome.

Diagnostics

An Allen test should be performed in all cases but has a reported sensitivity of 55% and specificity of 92%.[62] Other noninvasive tests include pulse volume recording, and plethysmography to evaluate for flow abnormalities. Ultrasonography or Doppler mapping can evaluate the ulnar artery for evidence of occlusion or compromised blood flow and the presence of a mural thrombus.[63] Contrast angiography is still considered the gold standard for diagnosis and allows excellent visualization of the vascular anatomy,[60] but has a 1% to 2% morbidity because of the need for intra-arterial catheterization and contrast infusion (**Fig. 8**). In addition to being helpful in the diagnosis, it may be a vehicle for intra-arterial thrombolysis, if indicated.[43,64] These modalities can be helpful for cases in which vascular reconstruction is not possible or to provide proximal or distal vessel patency before surgical reconstruction of a wrist or palm arterial defect.[43,64] Review of real-time sequential images greatly enhances surgeons' ability to estimate the extent of thrombosis and the quality of collateral flow, especially intraoperatively.[43,64] Computed tomographic angiography (sensitivity, 90%–95%; specificity, 98%–100%) and magnetic resonance angiography can be used in addition to contrast angiography. Apart from visualizing associated bone and muscle anatomy, these techniques are particularly useful in the setting of ulnar artery occlusions in determining whether the occlusion is also associated with ulnar artery aneurysmal dilatation.[35,43,61,65]

Non-Operative Treatment

Studies examining treatment outcomes of HHS in athletes are limited to case reports and small case series, and no consensus exists on best management practices.[35,61] Several conservative and surgical treatment options exist that may be tailored to the athlete in question. Although avoidance of repetitive trauma may not be an option for high-performing athletes, equipment modification may limit the exposure to trauma. For example, catcher mitts may be padded and modified to limit the impact of high-velocity pitches,[2] with custom-made padded gloves being used by ice hockey players.[43] Medical treatment may serve as a primary treatment strategy with vasodilators (eg, calcium channel blockers) and thrombolytics being the mainstay.[2,43] For example, athletes solely presenting with ulnar artery occlusions may not require immediate surgical exploration or revascularization.[60] Nonsurgical management of ulnar artery occlusions has similarly been reported through the use of selective catheter-directed intra-arterial thrombolytic therapy with successful ablation in patients with ischemic symptoms.[43,60,61,66,67] Other investigators have reported on the use of intra-arterial vasodilators.[68–71] Nuber and colleagues[72] treated 13 athletes from 1983 to 1988 (9 of whom were professional baseball catchers presenting with hand ischemia caused by HHS) nonoperatively with glove modification, cold avoidance, and optionally vasodilator infusions. Two patients presented with severe ischemia as well as continuous pain and were successfully treated with papaverine chloride infusion followed by intravenous heparin and dextran. All patients returned to their sports with resolution of symptoms.

Surgical Treatment

Surgical treatment may be pursued in the presence of symptomatic ischemia, vascular damage to multiple digital arteries with insufficient collateral circulation, or aneurysm formation.[73,74] Surgical strategies include ligation of the diseased ulnar artery, reverse vein reconstruction (eg, harvested from dorsum of the foot, or cephalic or basilic veins), or arterial interposition grafts (eg, harvested from inferior epigastric or lateral femoral circumflex) (**Figs. 9** and **10**). Advocates for arterial grafts claim improved long-term patency rates compared with venous grafts and better diameter/tapering matching.[75] Although a preference for arterial grafts is in line with cardiac surgery literature, long-term literature is lacking on grafting for the ulnar artery.[64]

Ligation of the involved segment of the ulnar artery prevents distal embolic events, eliminates the painful mass, relieves ulnar nerve compression, and removes the thrombus that initiated the vasospasm reflex.[76,77] Ligation requires proven adequate collateral circulation with a digital brachial index of 0.7 or more.[74,78,79] Larsen and colleagues[80] evaluated 75 cases of HHS over a 25-year period. The cohort consisted of 73 primary procedures and 2 resections for recurrent disease, and included (1) reconstruction using autologous great saphenous, cephalic, or other vein grafting in 61 arteries; (2) simple ligation in 8 patients; or (3) primary end-to-end anastomosis in 6 patients. The mean length of the diseased ulnar arteries was 4.2 ± 2.8 cm. Follow-up was available in 66 patients with a mean of 19.8 months and a median of 3.2 months. Complete resolution of symptoms was reported in 28 patients (42% of patients; 32 arteries). Significant improvement in symptoms was reported in an additional 34 patients (52% of patients; 38 arteries), and 4 patients (6% of patients; 4 arteries) reported no improvement. Persistent postoperative symptoms, based on 42 arteries, included cold intolerance (62%), pain (26%), tingling (17%), numbness (10%), and cyanosis (5%). Of the 62 patients who showed resolution or significant improvement, 5 (8%) presented later with recurrent severe symptoms and ulnar artery reocclusion (median, 2 years after initial repair; range, 1.5 months to 8 years). Two of these 5 patients underwent additional ulnar artery resections with vein grafting, both reporting complete resolution of symptoms after the second operation. The third underwent simple ligation of the ulnar artery, and the fourth sympathectomy, and both reported no symptomatic improvement. The last patient did not undergo additional surgical intervention.

Ferris and colleagues[37] reported good outcomes in 21 men with HHS, including 19 undergoing ulnar artery resections and reversed saphenous vein interposition grafting, 1 end-to-end anastomosis, and 1 ligation. At an average follow-up of 22 months (1–66 months) no recurrence of symptoms or signs was found in 16 of 19 patients with interposition grafts (84.2%), whereas in 3 patients late graft occlusion occurred. Lifchez and Higgins[74] reported on 14 cases of HHS, 2 of which were treated with direct ulnar artery repair, and the remaining 12 with venous grafts. After a mean follow-up of 52 months, all patients reported improvement in digital brachial index (0.82 vs 0.70), decrease in pain and dysesthesia, and a decrease in cold intolerance compared with preoperative values. The investigators reported a final patency rate of

Table 1
Overview of the literature for athletes with HHS

Author, Year	Gender	Age (y)	Sport	Side	Occlusion	Aneurysm	Intervention	Follow-up	Outcome
Conn et al,[31] 1970	Male	—	Karate	Right	—	—	Sympathectomy	—	—
Weeks and Young,[45] 1982	Male	27	Softball	Right	Yes	Yes	Primary: resection. Revision: venous grafting	—	Without symptoms at follow-up
Kostianen and Orava,[47] 1983	Male	17, 28, 25	Volleyball	Right	Yes	No	Conservative	4–8 mo	Full return to play without symptoms
Porubsky et al,[41] 1986	—	—	Hockey	—	Yes	—	Venous graft	—	Without symptoms at follow-up
McCarthy et al,[18] 1989	Male	—	Baseball/softball	—	Yes	—	Conservative	—	Full return to play without symptoms
	Male	—	Frisbee	—	Yes	—	Conservative	—	Full return to play without symptoms
De Monaco et al,[53] 1991	Male	29	Hockey	—	—	—	—	—	—
Koga et al,[50] 1993	Female	16	Badminton	Right	Yes	Yes	Venous graft	7 y	Full return to play without symptoms
Applegate and Spiegel,[56] 1995	Male	24, 37	Cycling	1: right. 2, left	Yes	—	1: conservative. 2: venous graft	—	2: after 1 mo graft occlusion
Schneider et al,[59] 1995	Male	31	Weight lifting	Right	Yes	No	Conservative	—	—

Study	Sex	Age	Sport	Side			Treatment	Follow-up	Outcome
Nakamura et al,[54] 1996	Female	55	Tennis	Right	Yes	Yes	End-to-end anastomosis	6 mo	Full return to amateur play
Müller et al,[49] 1997	Male	34	Golf	Left	Yes	Yes	Venous graft	—	—
Rowan,[44] 1998	Male	23	Baseball/softball	Right	Yes	No	Conservative with vasodilators intra-arterially	2 y	Reduced activity recreational level
Schneider et al,[51] 2002	Male	16	Breakdancing	Left	Yes	No	Thrombolysis	6 mo	Full return to play without symptoms
Rtaimate et al,[57] 2002	Male	20	Cycling	Left	Yes	Yes	Venous graft	3 y	Full return to play without symptoms
Galati et al,[52] 2003	Male	16	Soccer	Right	Yes	Yes	Ligation	1 y	Full return to play without symptoms
Cohen-Kashi et al,[46] 2012	Male	33	Basketball	Right	No	Yes	End-to-end anastomosis	3 y	Full return to amateur play
Zayed et al,[43] 2013	Male	26	Ice hockey	Right	Yes	No	Thrombolysis	3 mo	Full return to play without symptoms

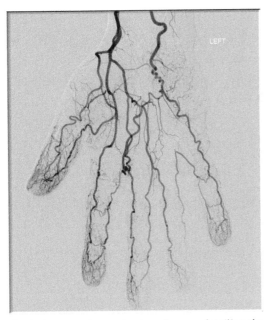

Fig. 8. Preoperative contrast angiogram detailing the tortuous course of the ulnar artery within the Guyon canal.

67%% (8 of 12). Patients who had developed ulnar artery occlusion had a better digital brachial index (0.19 vs 0.03) and greater subjective improvement in symptoms and function than those whose ulnar arteries remained patent. The investigators suggested that in these patients collateral flow may have developed and resulted in improved symptoms.

Dethmers and Houpt[73] evaluated the patency rate of saphenous vein grafts, arterial interposition grafts, and end-to-end anastomoses by duplex sonography in 27 cases with a mean follow-up period of 43 months (4–60 months). For vein grafts 4 cm or shorter, the grafts were patent in 5 patients, aneurysmal in 5, partially occluded in 1, and coiled in 1. In 8 venous interposition grafts that were 7 cm or longer, 5 of 8 were occluded.

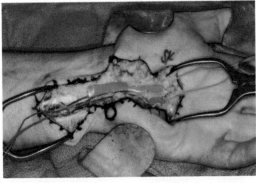

Fig. 9. Intraoperative view of diseased ulnar artery.

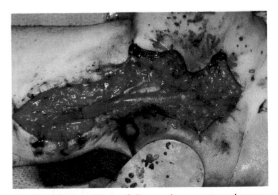

Fig. 10. After excision of diseased segment and reconstruction with reversed saphenous vein graft.

In 3 cases the investigators used arterial bypass grafts (the lateral femoral circumflex artery and thoracodorsal artery). The investigators found persistent mild to severe Raynaud phenomena in most of the operated hands, irrespective of the duplex sonography results. Patients treated with arterial grafts remained patent at follow-up. By comparison, only 8 of 24 venous grafts were fully patent.

Masden and colleagues[81] performed a comprehensive systematic review of grafting procedures for disorders of the distal upper extremity arterial vasculature. There were statistically significant improved patency rate for arterial grafts compared with vein grafts. Nineteen arterial grafts showed a patency of 100% at a mean follow-up of 18 months compared with an 85% patency rate of 133 vein grafts over 37 months. Within this cohort of patients, 112 patients with HHS were treated with vein grafts (patency of 82% at an average follow-up of 40%) compared with 13 arterial grafts (patency of 100% at 21 months; $P = .005$).

DIGITAL ISCHEMIA

Similarly to HHS, primary digital ischemia may occur through repeated microvascular trauma, especially in throwing, catching, or hand-smashing athletes, and has been reported in volleyball (31% prevalence),[82,83] baseball,[18,84–87] handball players,[88] as well as in karate.[89,90]

At the level of the metacarpal head, the neurovascular bundles are particularly susceptible to trauma, and may cause digital weakness, paresthesias, or pain.[91] Both the vibrational impact from catching balls thrown at high velocities and sympathetic hyperstimulation have been implicated as causes for microvascular occlusions distal to the level of the proximal interphalangeal joint.[85] In the throwing hand, vasculature may be compromised secondarily to hypertrophy of lumbrical muscles or Cleland ligaments.[87]

Because similar symptoms can occur in both vascular and neurologic disorders, thorough examination and accurate diagnoses are key. Symptoms closely parallel those of HHS, which may include digital ischemia and necrosis. The index finger is most often affected and may be as much as 4°C colder than its contralateral counterpart.[2] Conservative treatment includes rest and enhancement of protective equipment. Pharmacologic intervention is patient and disorder specific and may include thrombolytics, vasodilators (calcium channel blockers, topical nitroglycerin), or sympatholytic agents.[92] Itoh and colleagues[87] found a recurrence of symptoms on returning to play in elite baseball pitchers who were treated conservatively, and postulated proximal interphalangeal joint hyperextension and hypertrophy of Cleland ligaments as the cause of impingement, for which they performed a surgical release. In elite baseball players, decompression of the lumbrical canal allowed return to play within months in patients with occlusions of the first and second intermetacarpal arteries.[87]

SUMMARY

Impingement of neurovascular structures in the upper extremity can occur at many levels in athletes and can be caused by direct blunt trauma, an increased functional range, congenital or traumatic bony abnormalities, muscle hypertrophy, and joint translations. Impingements may lead to venous occlusions, arterial lesions, or aneurysmal degeneration causing secondary emboli, ischemia, and necrosis. Clinical symptoms often mimic common musculoskeletal injuries, making it difficult to diagnose the vascular cause of the disorders. Initial conservative treatment consists of avoidance of causative factors, careful inspection of equipment, enhancement of protective gear, and medical treatment using calcium canal blockers as well as thrombolytics. Although these measures are successful in most athletes and allow return to sport within several months without return of symptoms, some require surgical management. In these patients, thoracic outlet decompression, selective vessel ligation, or resection and reconstruction may allow a return to full activities without symptoms postoperatively within several months.

REFERENCES

1. Dillman CJ, Fleisig GS, Andrews JR. Biomechanics of pitching with emphasis upon shoulder kinematics. J Orthop Sports Phys Ther 1993;18:402–8.

2. Dugas JR, Weiland AJ. Vascular pathology in the throwing athlete. Hand Clin 2000;16:477–85.

3. Taylor AJ, George KP. Exercise induced leg pain in young athletes misdiagnosed as pain of musculoskeletal origin. Man Ther 2001;6:48–52.

4. Mosley JG. Arterial problems in athletes. Br J Surg 2003;90:1461–9.

5. Jackson MR. Upper extremity arterial injuries in athletes. Semin Vasc Surg 2003;16:232–9.

6. Arko FR, Harris EJ, Zarins CK, et al. Vascular complications in high-performance athletes. J Vasc Surg 2001;33:935–42.

7. Cahill BR, Palmer RE. Quadrilateral space syndrome. J Hand Surg Am 1983;8:65–9.

8. Reeser JC. Diagnosis and management of vascular injuries in the shoulder girdle of the overhead athlete. Curr Sports Med Rep 2007;6:322–7.

9. Nijhuis HH, Müller-Wiefel H. Occlusion of the brachial artery by thrombus dislodged from a traumatic aneurysm of the anterior humeral circumflex artery. J Vasc Surg 1991;13:408–11.

10. Reekers JA, den Hartog BM, Kuyper CF, et al. Traumatic aneurysm of the posterior circumflex humeral artery: a volleyball player's disease? J Vasc Interv Radiol 1993;4:405–8.

11. Durham JR, Yao JS, Pearce WH, et al. Arterial injuries in the thoracic outlet syndrome. J Vasc Surg 1995;21:57–70.

12. Hoskins WT, Pollard HP, McDonald AJ. Quadrilateral space syndrome: a case study and review of the literature. Br J Sports Med 2005;39:e9.

13. Duralde XA. Neurologic injuries in the athlete's shoulder. J Athl Train 2000;35:316–28.

14. McAdams TR, Dillingham MF. Surgical decompression of the quadrilateral space in overhead athletes. Am J Sports Med 2008;36:528–32.

15. Atema JJ, Unlü C, Reekers JA, et al. Posterior circumflex humeral artery injury with distal embolisation in professional volleyball players: a discussion of three cases. Eur J Vasc Endovasc Surg 2012;44:195–8.

16. Fleisig GS, Barrentine SW, Escamilla RF, et al. Biomechanics of overhand throwing with implications for injuries. Sports Med 1996;21:421–37.

17. Rohrer MJ, Cardullo PA, Pappas AM, et al. Axillary artery compression and thrombosis in throwing athletes. J Vasc Surg 1990;11:761–8 [discussion: 768–9].

18. McCarthy WJ, Yao JS, Schafer MF, et al. Upper extremity arterial injury in athletes. J Vasc Surg 1989;9:317–27.

19. Duwayri YM, Emery VB, Driskill MR, et al. Positional compression of the axillary artery causing upper extremity thrombosis and embolism in the elite overhead throwing athlete. J Vasc Surg 2011;53:1329–40.

20. Urschel HC Jr, Patel AN. Surgery remains the most effective treatment for Paget-Schroetter syndrome: 50 years' experience. Ann Thorac Surg 2008;86:254–60 [discussion: 260].

21. Sellke FW, Kelly TR. Thoracic outlet syndrome. Am J Surg 1988;156:54–7.

22. Feugier P, Aleksic I, Salari R, et al. Long-term results of venous revascularization for Paget-Schroetter syndrome in athletes. Ann Vasc Surg 2001;15:212–8.

23. Lee JT, Karwowski JK, Harris EJ, et al. Long-term thrombotic recurrence after nonoperative management of Paget-Schroetter syndrome. J Vasc Surg 2006;43:1236–43.

24. Fields WS, Lemak NA, Ben-Menachem Y. Thoracic outlet syndrome: review and reference to stroke in a major league pitcher. Am J Roentgenol 1986;146:809–14.

25. Casey RG, Richards S, ODonohoe M. Exercise induced critical ischaemia of the upper limb secondary to a cervical rib. Br J Sports Med 2003;37:455–6.

26. Cormier JM, Amrane M, Ward A, et al. Arterial complications of the thoracic outlet syndrome: fifty-five operative cases. J Vasc Surg 1989;9:778–87.

27. Paget J. On gouty and some other forms of phlebitis. St Bartholomews Hosp Rep 1866;82–92.

28. SL von Schroetter, Erkrankungen der Gefasse. Nathnagel Handbuch der Pathologie und Therapie. Holder, Wein (1884).

29. Hughes ES. Venous obstruction in the upper extremity; Paget-Schroetter's syndrome; a review of 320 cases. Surg Gynecol Obstet 1949;88:89–127.

30. Rutherford RB. Vascular surgery. Philadelphia: Saunders ; 2005. p. 1559–65.

31. Conn J Jr, Bergan JJ, Bell JL. Hypothenar hammer syndrome: posttraumatic digital ischemia. Surgery 1970;68:1122–8.

32. Von Rosen S. Ein Fall von Thrombose in der Arteria ulnaris nach Einwirkung von stumpfer Gewalt. Acta Chir Scand 1934;500–6.

33. Gross MS, Gelberman RH. The anatomy of the distal ulnar tunnel. Clin Orthop Relat Res 1985;(196):238–47.

34. Stone JR. Intimal hyperplasia in the distal ulnar artery: Influence of gender and implications for the hypothenar hammer syndrome. Cardiovasc Pathol 2004;13:20–5.

35. Ablett CT, Hackett LA. Hypothenar hammer syndrome: case reports and brief review. Clin Med Res 2008;6:3–8.

36. McClinton MA. Reconstruction for ulnar artery aneurysm at the wrist. J Hand Surg Am 2011;36:328–32.

37. Ferris BL, Taylor LM Jr, Oyama K, et al. Hypothenar hammer syndrome: proposed etiology. J Vasc Surg 2000;31:104–13.

38. Blum AG, Zabel JP, Kohlmann R, et al. Pathologic conditions of the hypothenar eminence: evaluation with multidetector CT and MR imaging. Radiographics 2006;26:1021–44.

39. Omokawa S, Tanaka Y, Ryu J, et al. Anatomy of the ulnar artery as it relates to the transverse carpal ligament. J Hand Surg Am 2002;27:101–4.

40. Netscher D, Polsen C, Thornby J, et al. Anatomic delineation of the ulnar nerve and ulnar artery in relation to the carpal tunnel by axial magnetic resonance imaging scanning. J Hand Surg Am 1996;21:273–6.

41. Porubsky GL, Brown SI, Urbaniak JR. Ulnar artery thrombosis: a sports-related injury. Am J Sports Med 1986;14:170–5.

42. Müller LP, Rudig L, Kreitner KF, et al. Hypothenar hammer syndrome in sports. Knee Surg Sports Traumatol Arthrosc 1996;4:167–70.

43. Zayed MA, McDonald J, Tittley JG. Hypothenar hammer syndrome from ice hockey stick-handling. Ann Vasc Surg 2013;27:1183.e5–10.

44. Rowan LJ. Hand ischemia in active patients: detecting and treating hypothenar hammer syndrome. Phys Sportsmed 1998;26:57–67.

45. Weeks PM, Young VL. Ulnar artery thrombosis and ulnar nerve compression associated with an anomalous hypothenar muscle. Plast Reconstr Surg 1982;69:130–1.

46. Cohen-Kashi KJ, Leeman J, Rothkopf I, et al. Traumatic ulnar artery aneurysm secondary to basketball dunk: a case report and review. Vascular 2012;20:96–9.

47. Kostianen S, Orava S. Blunt injury of the radial and ulnar arteries in volley ball players. A report of three cases of the antebrachial-palmar hammer syndrome. Br J Sports Med 1983;17:172–6.

48. Kleinert HE, Volianitis GJ. Thrombosis of the palmar arterial arch and its tributaries: etiology and newer concepts in treatment. J Trauma 1965;5:447–57.

49. Müller LP, Kreitner KF, Seidl C, et al. Traumatic thrombosis of the distal ulnar artery (hypothenar hammer syndrome) in a golf player with an accessory muscle loop around Guyon's canal. Handchir Mikrochir Plast Chir 1997;29:183–6.

50. Koga Y, Seki T, Caro LD. Hypothenar hammer syndrome in a young female badminton player. A case report. Am J Sports Med 1993;21:890–2.

51. Schneider F, Milesi I, Haesler E, et al. Break-dance: an unusual cause of hammer syndrome. Cardiovasc Intervent Radiol 2002;25:330–1.

52. Galati G, Cosenza UM, Sammartino F, et al. True aneurysm of the ulnar artery in a soccer goalkeeper: a case report and surgical considerations. Am J Sports Med 2003;31:457–8.

53. De Monaco D, Fritsche E, Rigoni G, et al. Hypothenar hammer syndrome: retrospective study of nine cases. J Hand Surg Br 1991;24:731–4.

54. Nakamura T, Kambayashi J, Kawasaki T, et al. Hypothenar hammer syndrome caused by playing tennis. Eur J Vasc Endovasc Surg 1996;11: 240–2.

55. Noël B, Hayoz D. A tennis player with hand claudication. Vasa 2000;29(2):151–3.

56. Applegate KE, Spiegel PK. Ulnar artery occlusion in mountain bikers. J Sports Med Phys Fitness 1995;35:232–4.

57. Rtaimate M, Farez E, Larivière J, et al. Anuerysm of the ulnar artery in a mountain biker. A case report and review of the literature. Chir Main 2002;21: 362–5.

58. Vanmaele RG, Van Schil PE, Van den Brande F, et al. Hypothenar snowboard syndrome. Eur J Vasc Endovasc Surg 1998;16:82–4.

59. Schneider M, Creutzig A, Alexander K. Traumatically-induced ischemia of the hands. Med Klin (Munich) 1995;90:225–8.

60. Yuen JC, Wright E, Johnson LA, et al. Hypothenar hammer syndrome. Ann Plast Surg 2011;67: 429–38.

61. Marie I, Hervé F, Primard E, et al. Long-term follow-up of hypothenar hammer syndrome: a series of 47 patients. Medicine (Baltimore) 2007;86:334–43.

62. Kohonen M, Teerenhovi O, Terho T, et al. Is the Allen test reliable enough? Eur J Cardiothorac Surg 2007;32:902–5.

63. Allen G, Wilson D. Ultrasound of the upper limb: when to use it in athletes. Semin Musculoskelet Radiol 2012;16:280–5.

64. Higgins JP, McClinton MA. Vascular insufficiency of the upper extremity. J Hand Surg Am 2010;35: 1545–53.

65. Bogdan MA, Klein MB, Rubin GD, et al. CT angiography in complex upper extremity reconstruction. J Hand Surg Br 2004;29:465–9.

66. Komorowska-Timek E, Teruya TH, Abou-Zamzam AM Jr, et al. Treatment of radial and ulnar artery pseudoaneurysms using percutaneous thrombin injection. J Hand Surg Am 2004;29:936–42.

67. Semba CP, Murphy TP, Bakal CW, et al. Thrombolytic therapy with use of alteplase (rt-PA) in peripheral arterial occlusive disease: review of the clinical literature. The Advisory Panel. J Vasc Interv Radiol 2000;11:149–61.

68. Duncan W. Hypothenar hammer syndrome: an uncommon cause of digital ischemia. J Am Acad Dermatol 1996;34:880–3.

69. Sharma R, Ladd W, Chaisson G. Images in cardiovascular medicine: hypothenar hammer syndrome. Circulation 2002;105:1615–6.

70. Mori KW, Bookstein JJ, Heeney DJ. Selective intra-arterial streptokinase infusion; clinical and laboratory correlates. Radiology 1983;148:677–82.

71. Yabukov S, Nappi J, Candela R. Successful prolonged local infusion of urokinase for the hypothenar hammer syndrome. Cathet Cardiovasc Diagn 1993;29(4):301–3.

72. Nuber GW, McCarthy WJ, Yao JS, et al. Arterial abnormalities of the hand in athletes. Am J Sports Med 1990;18:520–3.

73. Dethmers RS, Houpt P. Surgical management of hypothenar and thenar hammer syndromes: a retrospective study of 31 instances in 28 patients. J Hand Surg Br 2005;30:419–23.

74. Lifchez SD, Higgins JP. Long-term results of surgical treatment for hypothenar hammer syndrome. Plast Reconstr Surg 2009;124:210–6.

75. Fabbrocini M, Fattouch K, Camporini G, et al. The descending branch of lateral femoral circumflex artery in arterial CABG: early and midterm results. Ann Thorac Surg 2003;75:1836–41.

76. Cooke RA. Hypothenar hammer syndrome: a discrete syndrome to be distinguished from hand-arm vibration syndrome. Occup Med (Lond) 2003; 53:320–4.

77. Zweig J, Lie KK, Posch JL, et al. Thrombosis of the ulnar artery following blunt trauma to the hand. J Bone Joint Surg Am 1969;51:1191–8.

78. Zimmerman NB, Zimmerman SI, McClinton MA, et al. Long-term recovery following surgical treatment for ulnar artery occlusion. J Hand Surg Am 1994;19(1):17–21.

79. Chloros GD, Lucas RM, Li Z, et al. Post-traumatic ulnar artery thrombosis: outcome of arterial reconstruction using reverse interpositional vein grafting at 2 years minimum follow-up. J Hand Surg Am 2008;33:932–40.

80. Larsen BT, Edwards WD, Jensen MH, et al. Surgical pathology of hypothenar hammer syndrome with new pathogenetic insights. Am J Surg Pathol 2013;37:1700–8.

81. Masden DL, Seruya M, Higgins JP. A systematic review of the outcomes of distal upper extremity bypass surgery with arterial and venous conduits. J Hand Surg Am 2012;37:2362–7.

82. van de Pol D, Kuijer PP, Langenhorst T, et al. High prevalence of self-reported symptoms of digital ischemia in elite male volleyball players in the Netherlands: a cross-sectional national survey. Am J Sports Med 2012;40:2296–302.

83. van de Pol D, Kuijer PP, Langenhorst T, et al. Risk factors associated with self-reported symptoms of digital ischemia in elite male volleyball players in the Netherlands. Scand J Med Sci Sports 2013; 24:e230–7.

84. Ginn TA, Smith AM, Snyder JR, et al. Vascular changes of the hand in professional baseball players with emphasis on digital ischemia in catchers. J Bone Joint Surg Am 2005;87:1464–9.

85. Sugawara M, Ogino T, Minami A, et al. Digital ischemia in baseball players. Am J Sports Med 1986;14:329–34.

86. Lowrey CW, Chadwick RO, Waltman EN. Digital vessel trauma from repetitive impact in baseball catchers. J Hand Surg Am 1976;1: 236–8.

87. Itoh Y, Wakano K, Takeda T, et al. Circulatory disturbances in the throwing hand of baseball pitchers. Am J Sports Med 1987;15:264–9.

88. Buckhout BC, Warner MA. Digital perfusion of handball players: effects of repeated ball impact on structures of the hand. Am J Sports Med 1980;8:206–7.

89. Nieman EA, Swann PG. Karate injuries. Br Med J 1971;23(5742):233.

90. Vayssairat M, Priollet P, Capron L, et al. Does karate injure blood vessels of the hand? Lancet 1984;1(8401):529.

91. Ruchselman DE, Lee SK. Neurovasculature injuries of the hand in athletes. Curr Orthop Pract 2009;20: 409–15.

92. Koman LA, Urbaniak JR. Ulnar artery insufficiency: a guide to treatment. J Hand Surg Am 1981;6:16–24.

Current Options for Treatment of Hypothenar Hammer Syndrome

Helen G. Hui-Chou, MD, Michael A. McClinton, MD*

KEYWORDS

- Hypothenar hammer syndrome • Ulnar artery thrombosis • Ulnar artery aneurysm
- Arterial aneurysm • Vein/artery grafting

KEY POINTS

- Arteriography with contrast remains the gold standard for diagnosis and evaluation.
- Predisposing factors include tobacco smoking, manual labor (using hand as a hammer on a daily basis, daily pressure to palm of hand, daily exposure to vibrating tools), dominant hand, and male gender.
- Medical management includes smoking cessation, calcium channel blockers (nifedipine), and prostaglandins.
- Indications for operative treatment include failure of conservative management and critical digital ischemia.
- Surgical management includes resection of abnormal segment with ligation of vessel or reconstruction with venous or arterial grafts.
- Long term evaluation of graft and vessel patency remains inconsistent with patient symptoms.

INTRODUCTION

Thrombosis of the ulnar artery (UA) secondary to blunt trauma of the hand was first described in 1934 by von Rosen in a 23-year-old factory worker who was successfully treated with excision of the thrombosed artery.[1] The UA at the wrist is the most common site of arterial aneurysms of the upper extremity because it is superficial and lies over the hook of the hamate. Hypothenar hammer syndrome (HHS) is a rare vascular disorder resulting from injury to the UA at the level of Guyon canal. Conn and colleagues[2] coined the term HHS in 1970 because it is classically seen in workers who repeatedly use the hypothenar eminence as a substitute for a hammer.

The incidence of HHS has been reported from 1.6% to 14% in manual laborers, craftsmen, and habitual hand hammerers owing to repetitive blunt trauma.[3–6] Although most commonly associated with hand-intensive laborers such as mechanics, construction workers, and auto body repair workers, the condition has been diagnosed in athletes. These athletes were engaged in recreational activities including golf, badminton, squash, mountain biking, weightlifting, martial arts, baseball, basketball, football, hockey, and tennis.[5,7–11] Patients can present with a history of either a single or multiple repetitive traumas to the hand at the hypothenar eminence.

RELEVANT ANATOMY AND PATHOPHYSIOLOGY

The UA passes beneath the volar carpal ligament in Guyon canal covered only by the palmaris brevis

Disclosures: The authors have no conflicts of interest to disclose.
The Curtis National Hand Center, MedStar Union Memorial Hospital, 3333 North Calvert Street, #200, Baltimore, MD 21218, USA
* Corresponding author. Care of Anne Mattson, The Curtis National Hand Center, Medstar Union Memorial Hospital, 3333 North Calvert Street, #200, Baltimore, MD 21218.
E-mail address: anne.mattson@medstar.net

Hand Clin 31 (2015) 53–62
http://dx.doi.org/10.1016/j.hcl.2014.09.005
0749-0712/15/$ – see front matter © 2015 Elsevier Inc. All rights reserved.

muscle, subcutaneous tissue, and skin. Beneath this unprotected 2-cm segment of UA lies the hook of the hamate bone against which the artery can be pounded by external forces. In addition, the dorsal branch of the UA tethers the main UA, preventing it from being displaced off the hook of hamate during traumatic episodes. Repetitive trauma and occasionally single acute episodes can damage the medial wall of the artery, leading to UA thrombosis, occlusion, distal embolization, and aneurysmal degeneration and expansion of the wall.

UA aneurysms can be true aneurysms with all 3 layers of the arterial wall expanded producing a fusiform or sometimes corkscrew configuration. False or pseudoaneurysms result from penetrating trauma to the UA. In this case, the intima is breached and bleeding occurs external to the artery, forming a hematoma. Because this hematoma is connected to the UA, it may recannulize and form an eccentric fibrous outpouching of the artery without the 3 layers of the arterial wall. Pseudoaneurysms have a lower propensity for distal embolization, but they can expand and rupture, causing external bleeding.

Arterial injury may cause thrombosis and occlusion distal to the segment overlying the hamate bone extending into the superficial palmar arch and digital arteries. Damage to arterial wall media and elastic lamina results in an influx of platelets and macrophages to the site. Inflammatory mediators secreted by these cells stimulate hyperplasia, fibrosis, and thrombosis. Additionally, a mechanism of preexisting palmar UA fibrodysplasia has been proposed; despite the UA's vulnerable anatomic position, HHS has a relatively low incidence in the general population.[3,12] Thrombosis, segmental occlusion, and microemboli to the digital arteries may result in vascular insufficiency of the hand.

CLINICAL PRESENTATION AND EXAMINATION

Patients are predominantly male and present with symptoms of unilateral hand and digit ischemia, affecting the dominant hand most commonly (53%–93%).[5,13–16] Some cases of bilateral involvement have been reported.[17] Symptoms may be acute or chronic with recurrent episodes of pain, numbness, tingling, cold intolerance, and weakness in the ulnar nerve distribution. Symptoms vary depending on severity of occlusion and vascular insufficiency (**Fig. 1**).

On physical examination, the hand and ulnar digits, usually the long, ring, and small fingers, may have pallor, cyanosis, splinter hemorrhages, ulcerations, and/or wounds. Signs in the thumb have never been described.[15,18] A pulsatile mass may be found at the level of the wrist, with, at times, an absent pulse distal to the mass. **Table 1** lists signs and symptoms of HHS.

Several validated questionnaires have been designed in attempts to quantify the various symptoms and disabilities caused by hand ischemia.

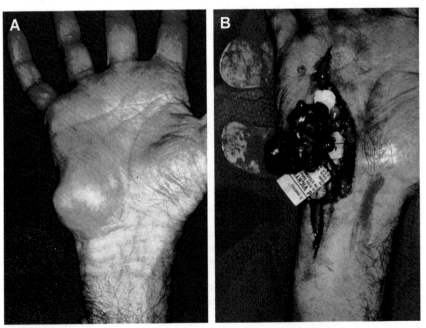

Fig. 1. Hypothenar pulsatile mass (*A*), which revealed an ulnar artery aneurysm (*B*).

Table 1
Symptoms and signs of hypothenar hammer syndrome

Symptoms	Signs
Pain	Pallor
Numbness	Cyanosis, mottling
Tingling	Palpable hypothenar mass
Cold intolerance	Atrophy of distal finger pads
Weakness in ulnar nerve distribution	Fingertip findings on long, ring, and small fingers: Splinter/subungal hemorrhages, ulcerations/wounds, gangrene

The Levine-Katz questionnaire assesses pain, dysesthesia symptoms, and hand function.[19,20] The McCabe Cold Sensitivity Test is a short and simple method to assess cold sensitivity and the complex array of symptoms patients often present.[21] Last, the Cold Intolerance Symptom Severity questionnaire was designed and validated to combine questions and assessments not addressed by the McCabe Cold Sensitivity Tests.[22–24] Any of these questionnaires can assist clinicians in quantifying symptoms as well has measuring improvement of symptoms after treatment.

Predisposing risk factors for HHS include tobacco smoking, strenuous manual labor (using the hand as a hammer on a daily basis, daily pressure to palm of the hand, daily exposure to vibrating tools), dominant hand, and male gender.[17] Important patient history includes the presence of other vascular disease, including metabolic and connective tissue disease, recreation risks factors, and living in a cold environment. Preexisting fibrodysplasia of the UA may also be a predisposing factor for HHS.[3,12]

DIAGNOSTIC PROCEDURES

Diagnostic testing is useful for screening or diagnosis of HHS. These procedures can be performed in the office setting, vascular laboratory, and separate imaging facilities. There are noninvasive, minimally invasive, and invasive procedures. Further diagnostic imaging allows determination of location, morphology, extent of vessel damage, and presence of collateral blood supply around the vascular obstruction.

In-office diagnostic testing is first performed to evaluate vascular insufficiency of the hand owing to HHS. The Allen test is typically positive, but sensitivity is only 55% and specificity is 92%.[25] A hand-held pencil Doppler may be used to determine the site of occlusion of the UA and presence of distal blood flow in the digits.

Noninvasive diagnostic testing is useful as a screening or diagnostic tool, especially for patients with chronic symptoms at presentation.[26,27] A pulse volume recording (PVR) is designed to measure the volume of arterial blood flow (circulation) and is easily performed, reproducible, and provides generated graphic wave forms on a chart for clinicians. PVR can detect inadequate arterial blood flow to the hand and digits by comparing proximal and distal blood flow. PVR can determine the presence, severity, and general location of peripheral arterial occlusive disease. The digital brachial index (DBI) quantifies abnormal perfusion to the hand and digits by comparing digital blood pressure with the contralateral brachial level blood pressure. The normal range for DBI is 0.75 to 0.97. When the DBI is equal or less than 0.7, perfusion is inadequate. Doppler ultrasonography (US) or vascular duplex US can measure blood flow through arteries and veins. This study provides audible flow information and color-coded images. Duplex US can demonstrate flow abnormalities, deficient UA flow, wall irregularity, echogenic intraluminal thrombus, and aneurysm in patients with HHS. Duplex US may show bidirectional color flow in aneurysms or pseudoaneurysms, providing detailed information on the extent and site of impaired blood flow. It is utilized as a screening tool in high-risk populations with concern for HHS. The disadvantage of a Duplex US is the lack of standardization and documentation, because the study is often performed at different locations or departments.[6,15,28–30] If any noninvasive tests are abnormal, the surgeon may proceed with further, more invasive diagnostic testing.

There are 2 minimally invasive diagnostic studies that provide more information and detail on the vasculature than PVR, DBI, or US. Computed tomographic angiography (CTA) and magnetic resonance angiography (MRA) are minimally invasive tests that require venous access for administration of a contrast dye. Both studies perform simultaneous evaluation of both hands, which allows comparative assessment of vascular architecture. CTA utilizes 3-dimensional formatting and offers details of anatomic relationships between bones, soft tissues, and the vascular system. CTA has a fast acquisition time and a lower dose of radiation exposure than conventional arteriography.[31] MRA provides similar anatomic details specifically for soft tissue architecture as the CTA. MRA requires administration of a contrast dye that is less nephrotoxic than CTA contrast dye.[32] However, MRA is highly susceptible to movement artifact owing to its long acquisition time and is contraindicated in patients with metallic implants and claustrophobia. Neither CTA nor MRA provides flow data.[29–33] A 2004 study by Bogdan and colleagues[31] noted the costs differential between these studies with US flow duplex at $450, CTA at $1140, MRA at $2500, and conventional angiography costing $3900.

Conventional angiography/arteriography remains the gold standard for evaluation of HHS.[3,29,34,35] Conventional angiography can demonstrate several pathognomonic features of HHS, including tortuosity of the UA leading to a "corkscrew appearance," with alternating stenosis and ectasia. Arteriography can also show aneurysm formation, occlusion of the UA segment overlying the hook of the hamate, occluded superficial palmar arch or digital arteries, with a normal proximal UA (**Fig. 2**). Evaluation of the arterial vasculature requires digital subtraction angiography. Digital subtraction angiography does not provide information regarding venous anatomy or soft tissue anatomic relationships. Conventional angiography requires arterial access for contrast dye administration. Risks include bleeding, hematoma, thrombosis, pseudoaneurysm, allergy to contrast medium, renal toxicity from contrast, and a dose of 4 times more radiation than CTA. Therefore, conventional angiography is not utilized as screening tool and is contraindicated in patients with renal insufficiency.

TREATMENT

HHS is a treatable condition; however, the appropriate treatment of the patient with HHS is not universally agreed on for each specific case. The goals of treatment are restoration of blood flow to the ischemic digits and prevention of further thrombotic or embolic sequelae. Optimal therapy for HHS has not been determined with controlled studies of the various treatment options. Treatment options for each patient may be limited by the extent of disease at presentation. Vascular insufficiency with ischemic symptoms and

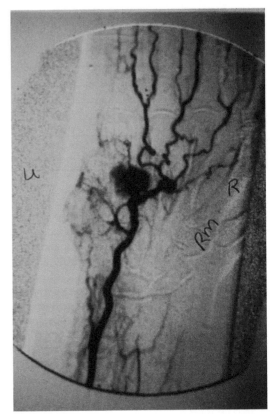

Fig. 2. Conventional angiography of ulnar artery aneurysm.

imminent tissue loss requires more aggressive nonoperative treatment and earlier operative management. Treatment options may vary with patient age, patient occupation, other medical comorbidities, and vascular disease.

Conservative treatment options are used for patients who are not at risk for impending tissue loss, necrosis, or active ischemia. Conservative and medical treatment options can be adjuncts to any surgical interventions attempted. Conservative management includes activity modification, smoking cessation, pain control, calcium channel blockers, α-blockers, β-blockers, and steroids. Intravenous and oral vasodilators, including prostaglandins and prostacyclin, have been used to decrease sympathetic tone and vasospasm.[5,36] The vasodilation effect as well as inhibition of platelet aggregation led to healing of digital ulcers in all the patients who were not surgical candidates in the series. With evidence of thrombosis and embolic disease, anticoagulation, and platelet aggregation inhibitors have been effective as both primary therapies and adjuncts preoperatively and postoperatively. Antiplatelet agents include clopidogrel and aspirin. Anticoagulation has been described with acute use of low-molecular-weight heparin, dextran, or heparin. Long-term anticoagulation can be continued with warfarin or low-molecular-weight heparin.[7]

Criteria for surgical intervention in patients include failure of medical management to relieve symptoms, failure of local treatment to heal any digital soft tissue problems, and presence of a reconstructable lesion on angiography or intraoperative assessment.[20] Surgical intervention can be characterized as either nonoperative intervention or direct open intravascular access.

Nonoperative treatment employs a percutaneous approach. One technique directs intra-arterial thrombolytics to the site of UA thrombosis. Catheter-directed thrombolytic administration with recombinant tissue plasminogen activator or urokinase can provide definitive treatment by clearing thrombosis and relieving symptoms. Success of this procedure may be limited if ischemic symptoms are severe or have persisted for more than 2 weeks.[4,32,37] Overall success rates of intra-arterial thrombolysis are 55% to 75%, with a 30% complication rate. Results seem to be inferior to surgery for more distal occlusions.[15,38] Intra-arterial thrombolysis can be utilized as preoperative therapy to decrease the amount of thrombosis before reconstruction of the artery, which improves success rates of 77% to 100%.[39] Complications of thrombolytic therapy include access site hematoma and generalized bleeding.

A case report of HHS being treated with percutaneous angioplasty of the distal radial artery was described in a patient who had occlusion of both radial and ulnar arteries at the wrist level. He was a poor surgical candidate and had already had partial digital amputations. Balloon angioplasty was able to open the occluded lumen and the patient had resolution of symptoms and healing of distal fingertip wounds. Although percutaneous angioplasty is well established for coronary, lower extremity, and proximal upper extremity vessels, it has not been well studied for patency in vessels distal to brachial artery bifurcation.[40]

Madaric and colleagues[41] described the use of autologous intra-arterial bone marrow infusion for a patient with HHS and single distal digit ischemia and necrosis. The patient was not a candidate for traditional treatment options. A 1-time intra-arterial infusion of autologous bone marrow was administered with resolution of rest pain symptoms, fingertip necrosis, and improved DBI.

Open operative treatment modalities include sympathectomy, exploration with ligation of diseased segment, exploration with excision and primary repair of UA, and exploration with revascularization procedure.

Sympathectomy can be performed at thoracic, cervical, or digital levels to decrease sympathetic tone to the affected extremity. Cervical and thoracic sympathectomies are not routinely done owing to postoperative side effects such as dry hands and reflex compensatory sweating. When initially described, they were used in conjunction with exploration and ligation of the distal UA.[11] Digital sympathectomy with botulinum toxin A has been described for treating vasospasm leading to improvement of digital ischemia. Chemical digital sympathectomy has low morbidity and is noninvasive. Most describe injection of 100 units of botulinum toxin A into the affected hand and digits; however, the most effective dosing is not known.[27,42–44]

A Leriche sympathectomy consists of ligation and excision of the diseased segment of UA. Von Rosen used this treatment in 1934.[1] Ligation is a viable option if critical ischemia is not identified preoperatively (DBI of 0.7 or less). With a normal DBI, the UA can be sacrificed because most patients are radial artery dominant.[13,26,45–47] UA ligation constitutes a local sympathectomy, aided by the division of the terminal branches of the nerve of Henle. The UA is sacrificed in other instances, such as with the ulnar forearm flap. This flap is often used in reconstructive surgery without reconstitution of the UA. Although these patients do not have upper extremity ischemia at presentation, loss of the UA did not cause development of any ischemic symptoms, or impairment of perfusion, sensation, or motor function.[48] UA ligation increases the risk for development of vascular insufficiency and ischemia in the future, especially in younger patients.

Early reports of operative management for HHS included exploration, excision of diseased segment, and primary repair of the UA.[13,49,50] This restored blood flow to the ischemic digits and was effective if there remained adequate vessel length after resection to allow primary anastomosis without tension across the repair. However, vascular disease of UA had often propagated proximally or distally, resulting in longer defects after resection.

Currently, the preferred method of operative management for HHS is exploration and revascularization of the UA.[4,13,26,27,49,51] There are 2 types of revascularization procedures. A bypass graft utilizes a proximal anastomosis and is performed end to side. The diseased segment of UA is preserved. The segment may be ligated to reduce the risk of further embolic sequelae. The bypass graft is sutured distally to superficial palmar arch or digital arteries. In theory, there is decreased operative time and a less extensive dissection if the disease segment is left in place (**Fig. 3**).[52,53] Revascularization is more commonly performed with an interposition graft. Here, the diseased segment of UA is excised and the interposition graft is inserted using an end-to-end technique from proximal healthy UA to distal targets. The distal anastomosis may be distal UA, superficial arch, or even common or proper digital arteries.

The revascularization procedure improves blood flow to the hand and digits and may restore normal flow on vascular testing. A donor vessel is needed to bridge the gap. Donor vessels can either be venous or arterial, and selection may depend on various factors. Vein interpositional grafts were used initially for revascularization procedures.[49,54] The presence of valves requires either the vein to be reversed before inset or a valvulotome must be used for anterograde flow through the vein. The advantages of using vein grafts are that they are more expendable than arterial grafts, available from multiple sites from the body, are often found in a superficial plane for harvest, and provide longer donor vessel lengths. Some disadvantages are the need to reverse or use valvulotome, size mismatch to distal branches

of the UA, and flimsy handling characteristics.[32] There are multiple donor sites for vein grafts from the arms, legs, and feet. **Table 2** provides detailed descriptions of donor grafts.

Arterial grafts are more physiologic conduits than vein grafts. Advantages of arterial grafts include more distal branching options to match normal arterial branching in the hand, ability to maintain their normal proximal-to-distal orientation, and better handling characteristics. Disadvantages of the artery include shorter lengths (<15–20 cm), fewer donor sites, and deeper planes of dissection for harvest.[55–58] Arterial conduits are listed in **Table 2**.

Arteries described for use as arterial conduit grafts include the subscapular, superficial and deep inferior epigastric, thoracodorsal, and lateral circumflex femoral arteries. The subscapular artery alone provides a very short pedicle and requires patient repositioning during surgery. The thoracodorsal artery can be harvested from the contralateral arm and therefore allows a 2-team approach. It provides a significantly longer pedicle, described as up to 14 cm. The inferior epigastric system provides a superficial and

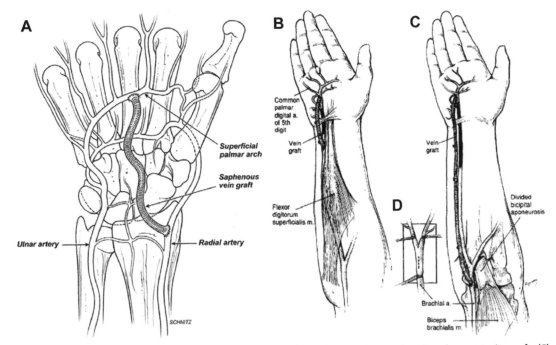

Fig. 3. (*A*) Bypass from the radial artery to the superficial palmar arch using a reversed saphenous vein graft. (*B*) Ulnar–ulnar vein bypass graft using forearm inflow. Note relationship to flexor digitorum superficialis muscle. a., artery; m., muscle. (*C*) Extensive forearm involvement may require inflow from the brachial artery just below the elbow. (*D*) The bicipital aponeurosis may need to be partially divided to optimize exposure. ([*A*] *From* Namdari S, Weiss AP, Carney WI. Palmar bypass for digital ischemia. J Hand Surg Am 2007;32(8):1252, with permission; and [*B–D*] Dalman RL. Upper extremity arterial bypass distal to the wrist. Ann Vasc Surg 1997;11(5):553, with permission.)

Table 2
Donor grafts

Graft	Length (cm)	Size Match for UA	Advantage	Disadvantage
Vein				
Greater saphenous	50–85	Poor	Found in superficial plane, longer lengths, easier dissection and harvest	Must be reversed or use valvulotome, decreased patency long-term, flimsy handling characteristics
Lesser saphenous	35–60	Good		
Forearm	14–20	Good		
Basilic/cephalic	15–30	Poor		
Dorsum foot	5–8	Good		
Artery				
Subscapular	2–4	Good	Improved patency rates, better size match, more distal branching options, easier to suture artery	Short pedicle length
Superficial inferior epigastric	6–10	Good		Abdominal bulge
Deep inferior epigastric	10–12	Good		Abdominal bulge, may be ligated during cesarean section
Thoracodorsal	11–14	Good		Dissection in axilla
Lateral circumflex femoral	10–18	Good, 2–5 mm		Deep, variable anatomy

deep branch. Typically, one of these is used as an arterial conduit. If a patient has a cesarean section scar, the inferior epigastric system may have been previously ligated. The superficial inferior epigastric artery can provide a 6-cm arterial graft, but it is absent in 35% of patients. The deep inferior epigastric artery can provide lengths of up to 12 cm, but its harvest can cause weakening of the rectus abdominis muscle and risk for abdominal bulge or herniation.[57,58]

The descending branch of the lateral circumflex femoral artery is our preferred arterial conduit for UA revascularization. Lengths of up to 19 cm have been harvested with a distal branching pattern that matches proper digital vessel branching in the hand. The lateral circumflex femoral artery is relatively easy to harvest located between the rectus femoris and vastus lateralis muscles. It has a comparable size match to the UA. Complications include numbness after transection of distal branches of the lateral femoral cutaneous nerve, neuroma formation, and hypertrophic scar formation.[57,59]

CLINICAL OUTCOMES IN THE LITERATURE

Treatment outcomes vary with management options. Ideally, there should be restoration of distal flow with resolution of rest pain and ischemic symptoms. However, short- and long-term results are often determined by patient factors, and not just the specific treatment. Most patients with HHS have persistent symptoms, although with lessened frequency and severity. Short-term complications after operative treatment include persistent cold intolerance, thrombosis of the graft, donor site complications (neuroma), wound healing complications, and stiffness of hand.[60] Marie and colleagues[5] reviewed a series of 47 patients and found that HSS recurrence was 27.7% after treatment with conservative medical management. Surgical treatment resulted in the healing of digital necrosis, with no recurrence of HHS. With these patients, 69.2% continued smoking and 80% continued occupational exposure to repetitive hand trauma.

Operative intervention with revascularization has the highest rate of improvement of ischemic symptoms with decreased pain. Studies have further measured outcomes of surgical revascularization by long-term follow-up of vessel patency in both venous and arterial grafts. Arterial grafts show consistently higher rates of long-term patency; however, venous grafts patency is acceptable, at 77% to 88% in most series.[3,5,11,47,54,61] Masden and colleagues[62] performed a systematic review of the literature, which demonstrated a higher patency rate and clinical efficacy of upper extremity bypass with arterial conduits with almost a 3-year follow-up when compared with venous conduits. Longer vein conduits also had a lower patency rate at long-term follow-up.[11,55] Arterial conduits may be ideal for revascularization of UA in the younger and active patient populations. Regardless of graft patency, patients seem to have the highest rate of relief of ischemic symptoms and improvement of DBI after surgical revascularization procedures.

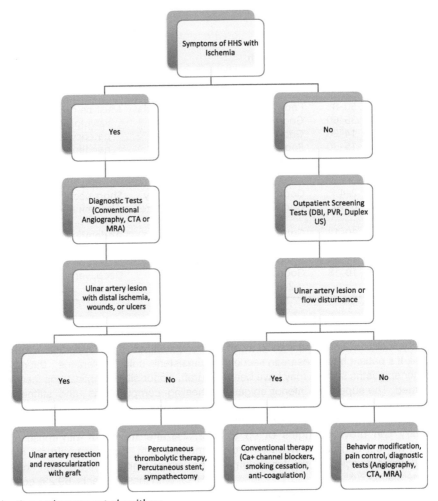

Fig. 4. Evaluation and treatment algorithms.

SUMMARY

HHS is a rare vascular condition resulting from acute or chronic injury to a 2-cm segment of the UA. Patients may be asymptomatic or present with acute or chronic episodes of ischemic symptoms. **Fig. 4** provides a summary of evaluation and treatment algorithms. Conventional angiography remains the gold standard in diagnosis of HHS. Treatment options are selected based on the severity of the patient's presenting symptoms. Management may include medical therapy, interventional procedures, and surgical intervention. Although no randomized studies have been performed on the efficacy of the treatment options, patients respond well to interventions with reported improvement of symptoms in multiple case series. Surgical exploration with resection

of the diseased UA and bypass with either a vein or artery interposition graft is our treatment option of choice.

REFERENCES

1. Von Rosen S. Ein fal von thrombose in der arteria ulnaris nach einwirkung von stumpfer gewald. Acta Chir Scand 1934;73:500–6.
2. Conn J Jr, Bergan JJ, Bell JL. Hypothenar hammer syndrome: posttraumatic digital ischemia. Surgery 1970;68(6):1122–8.
3. Ferris BL, Taylor LM Jr, Oyama K, et al. Hypothenar hammer syndrome: proposed etiology. J Vasc Surg 2000;31(1 Pt 1):104–13.
4. Yuen JC, Wright E, Johnson LA, et al. Hypothenar hammer syndrome: an update with algorithms for

diagnosis and treatment. Ann Plast Surg 2011; 67(4):429–38.

5. Marie I, Herve F, Primard E, et al. Long-term follow-up of hypothenar hammer syndrome: a series of 47 patients. Medicine (Baltimore) 2007;86(6):334–43.

6. Little JM, Ferguson DA. The incidence of the hypothenar hammer syndrome. Arch Surg 1972; 105(5):684–5.

7. Zayed MA, McDonald J, Tittley JG. Hypothenar hammer syndrome from ice hockey stick-handling. Ann Vasc Surg 2013;27(8):1183.e5–10.

8. Nakamura T, Kambayashi J, Kawasaki T, et al. Hypothenar hammer syndrome caused by playing tennis. Eur J Vasc Endovasc Surg 1996;11(2):240–2.

9. Cohen-Kashi KJ, Leeman J, Rothkopf I, et al. Traumatic ulnar artery aneurysm secondary to basketball dunk: a case report and review. Vascular 2012;20(2):96–9.

10. Nitecki S, Anekstein Y, Karram T, et al. Hypothenar hammer syndrome: apropos of six cases and review of the literature. Vascular 2008;16(5):279–82.

11. Dethmers RS, Houpt P. Surgical management of hypothenar and thenar hammer syndromes: a retrospective study of 31 instances in 28 patients. J Hand Surg Br 2005;30(4):419–23.

12. Stone JR. Intimal hyperplasia in the distal ulnar artery; Influence of gender and implications for the hypothenar hammer syndrome. Cardiovasc Pathol 2004;13(1):20–5.

13. Koman LA, Urbaniak JR. Ulnar artery insufficiency: a guide to treatment. J Hand Surg Am 1981;6(1): 16–24.

14. Benedict KT Jr, Chang W, McCready FJ. The hypothenar hammer syndrome. Radiology 1974; 111(1):57–60.

15. Pineda CJ, Weisman MH, Bookstein JJ, et al. Hypothenar hammer syndrome. Form of reversible Raynaud's phenomenon. Am J Med 1985;79(5): 561–70.

16. Carpentier PH, Biro C, Jiguet M, et al. Prevalence, risk factors, and clinical correlates of ulnar artery occlusion in the general population. J Vasc Surg 2009;50(6):1333–9.

17. Scharnbacher J, Claus M, Reichert J, et al. Hypothenar hammer syndrome: a multicenter case-control study. Am J Ind Med 2013;56(11):1352–8.

18. Larsen BT, Edwards WD, Jensen MH, et al. Surgical pathology of hypothenar hammer syndrome with new pathogenetic insights: a 25-year institutional experience with clinical and pathologic review of 67 cases. Am J Surg Pathol 2013; 37(11):1700–8.

19. Levine DW, Simmons BP, Koris MJ, et al. A self-administered questionnaire for the assessment of severity of symptoms and functional status in carpal tunnel syndrome. J Bone Joint Surg Am 1993; 75A(11):1585–92.

20. Lifchez SD, Higgins JP. Long-term results of surgical treatment for hypothenar hammer syndrome. Plast Reconstr Surg 2009;124(1):210–6.

21. McCabe SJ, Mizgala C, Glickman L. The measurement of cold sensitivity of the hand. J Hand Surg 1991;16A(6):1037–40.

22. Irwin MS, Gilbert SE, Terenghi G, et al. Cold intolerance following peripheral nerve injury. Natural history and factors predicting severity of symptoms. J Hand Surg Br 1997;22(3):308–16.

23. Ruijs AC, Jaquet JB, Daanen HA, et al. Cold intolerance of the hand measured by the CISS questionnaire in a normative study population. J Hand Surg Br 2006;31(5):533–6.

24. Carlsson I, Cederlund R, Hoglund P, et al. Hand injuries and cold sensitivity: reliability and validity of cold sensitivity questionnaires. Disabil Rehabil 2008;30(25):1920–8.

25. Kohonen M, Teerenhovi O, Terho T, et al. Is the Allen test reliable enough? Eur J Cardiothorac Surg 2007;32(6):902–5.

26. Netscher DT, Janz B. Treatment of symptomatic ulnar artery occlusion. J Hand Surg 2008;33A(9): 1628–31.

27. Higgins JP, McClinton MA. Vascular insufficiency of the upper extremity. J Hand Surg 2010;35A: 1545–53.

28. Coulier B, Goffin D, Malbecq S, et al. Colour duplex sonographic and multislice spiral CT angiographic diagnosis of ulnar artery aneurysm in hypothenar hammer syndrome. JBR-BTR 2003;86(4):211–4.

29. Dreizin D, Jose J. Hypothenar hammer syndrome. Am J Orthop (Belle Mead NJ) 2012;41(8):380–2.

30. Gimenez DC, Gilabert OV, Ruiz JG, et al. Ultrasound and magnetic resonance angiography features of post-traumatic ulnar artery pseudoaneurysm: a case report and review of the literature. Skeletal Radiol 2009;38(9):929–32.

31. Bogdan MA, Klein MB, Rubin GD, et al. CT angiography in complex upper extremity reconstruction. J Hand Surg 2004;29B(5):465–9.

32. Buda SJ, Johanning JM. Brachial, radial, and ulnar arteries in the endovascular era: choice of intervention. Semin Vasc Surg 2005;18(4):191–5.

33. Winterer JT, Ghanem N, Roth M, et al. Diagnosis of the hypothenar hammer syndrome by high-resolution contrast-enhanced MR angiography. Eur Radiol 2002;12(10):2457–62.

34. Ablett CT, Hackett LA. Hypothenar hammer syndrome: case reports and brief review. Clin Med Res 2008;6(1):3–8.

35. Abdel-Gawad EA, Bonatti H, Housseini AM, et al. Hypothenar hammer syndrome in a computer programmer: CTA diagnosis and surgical and endovascular treatment. Vasc Endovascular Surg 2009;43(5):509–12.

36. Clifford PC, Martin MF, Sheddon EJ, et al. Treatment of vasospastic disease with prostaglandin E1. Br Med J 1980;281(6247):1031–4.

37. Bakhach J, Chahidi N, Conde A. Hypothenar hammer syndrome: management of distal embolization by intra-arterial fibrinolytics. Chir Main 1998;17(3):215–20.

38. Cejna M, Salomonowitz E, Wohlschlager H, et al. rt-PA thrombolysis in acute thromboembolic upper-extremity arterial occlusion. Cardiovasc Intervent Radiol 2001;24(4):218–23.

39. Katz SG, Kohl RD. Direct revascularization for the treatment of forearm and hand ischemia. Am J Surg 1993;165(3):312–6.

40. Namdari S, Park MJ, Weiss AP, et al. Chronic hand ischemia treated with radial artery balloon angioplasty: case report. J Hand Surg Am 2008;33(4):551–4.

41. Madaric J, Klepanec A, Mistrik M, et al. Intra-arterial autologous bone marrow cell transplantation in a patient with upper-extremity critical limb ischemia. Cardiovasc Intervent Radiol 2013;36(2):545–8.

42. Iorio ML, Masden DL, Higgins JP. Botulinum toxin A treatment of Raynaud's phenomenon: a review. Semin Arthritis Rheum 2012;41(4):599–603.

43. Neumeister MW, Chambers CB, Herron MS, et al. Botox therapy for ischemic digits. Plast Reconstr Surg 2009;124(1):191–201.

44. Neumeister MW. Botulinum toxin type A in the treatment of Raynaud's phenomenon. J Hand Surg Am 2010;35(12):2085–92.

45. Kleinert HE, Burget GC, Morgan JA, et al. Aneurysms of the hand. Arch Surg 1973;106(4):554–7.

46. Kleinert JM, Fleming SG, Abel CS, et al. Radial and ulnar artery dominance in normal digits. J Hand Surg 1989;14A(3):504–8.

47. Zimmerman NB, Zimmerman SI, McClinton MA, et al. Long-term recovery following surgical treatment for ulnar artery occlusion. J Hand Surg 1994;19A(1):17–21.

48. Brown EN, Chaudhry A, Mithani SK, et al. Long-term vascular, motor, and sensory donor site outcomes after ulnar forearm flap harvest. J Reconstr Microsurg 2014;30(2):115–20.

49. Given KS, Puckett CL, Kleinert HE. Ulnar artery thrombosis. Plast Reconstr Surg 1978;61(3):405–11.

50. Gelberman RH, Nunley JA, Koman LA, et al. The results of radial and ulnar arterial repair in the forearm. Experience in three medical centers. J Bone Joint Surg Am 1982;64(3):383–7.

51. Harris EJ Jr, Taylor LM Jr, Edwards JM, et al. Surgical treatment of distal ulnar artery aneurysm. Am J Surg 1990;159(5):527–30.

52. Dalman RL. Upper extremity arterial bypass distal to the wrist. Ann Vasc Surg 1997;11(5):550–7.

53. Namdari S, Weiss AP, Carney WI Jr. Palmar bypass for digital ischemia. J Hand Surg 2007;32A(8):1251–8.

54. Mehlhoff TL, Wood MB. Ulnar artery thrombosis and the role of interposition vein grafting: patency with microsurgical technique. J Hand Surg 1991;16A(2):274–8.

55. Leclere FM, Mordon S, Schoofs M. Acute digital ischemia: a neglected microsurgical emergency. Report of 17 patients and literature review. Microsurgery 2010;30(3):207–13.

56. McClinton MA. Reconstruction for ulnar artery aneurysm at the wrist. J Hand Surg 2011;36A(2):328–32.

57. Masden DL, McClinton MA. Arterial conduits for distal upper extremity bypass. J Hand Surg Am 2013;38(3):572–7.

58. Smith HE, Dirks M, Patterson RB. Hypothenar hammer syndrome: distal ulnar artery reconstruction with autologous inferior epigastric artery. J Vasc Surg 2004;40(6):1238–42.

59. Temming JF, van Uchelen JH, Tellier MA. Hypothenar hammer syndrome: distal ulnar artery reconstruction with autologous descending branch of the lateral circumflex femoral artery. Tech Hand Up Extrem Surg 2011;15(1):24–7.

60. Keo HH, Umer M, Baumgartner I, et al. Long-term clinical outcomes in patients diagnosed with severe digital ischemia. Swiss Med Wkly 2011;141:w13159.

61. Chloros GD, Lucas RM, Li Z, et al. Post-traumatic ulnar artery thrombosis: outcome of arterial reconstruction using reverse interpositional vein grafting at 2 years minimum follow-up. J Hand Surg Am 2008;33(6):932–40.

62. Masden DL, Seruya M, Higgins JP. A systematic review of the outcomes of distal upper extremity bypass surgery with arterial and venous conduits. J Hand Surg Am 2012;37(11):2362–7.

Connective Tissue Disorders Associated with Vasculitis and Vaso-Occlusive Disease of the Hand

Brett Michelotti, MD[a], Marco Rizzo, MD[b],
Steven L. Moran, MD[b],*

KEYWORDS

- Scleroderma • Lupus • Buerger disease • Hand ischemia • Hand vasculitis

KEY POINTS

- Vasospastic symptoms are common with scleroderma, systemic lupus erythematosus, and Buerger disease.
- Recent success with botulinum toxin injections has provided new hope for patients wishing to avoid surgery.
- If a patient fails medical management, distal sympathectomies in conjunction with vascular reconstruction can help in preventing tissue loss and preserving hand function.

INTRODUCTION

Vasculitis is a secondary finding in many autoimmune disease processes, including rheumatoid arthritis, scleroderma, and thyroiditis. Certain forms of vasculitis have a predilection for upper extremity involvement, and over time can lead to debilitating changes to the hand. Many of these conditions are now managed with tumor necrosis factor α regulators, which can prevent the development of occlusive disease, tissue ischemia, and tissue loss. Unfortunately, several disease conditions are still recalcitrant to many medications and can result in ischemic changes within the hand, which may require operative intervention. This article briefly reviews the major connective tissue disorders associated with vasculitis and vaso-occlusive disease of the hand, and their surgical treatment.

VASOSPASTIC AND VASO-OCCLUSIVE DISEASE

The body maintains tight regulatory control over the peripheral vasculature. Autonomic control of vasoconstriction and vasodilatation allows for a balance of adequate nutritional flow and thermoregulatory control, and prevents blood loss in the setting of trauma. Dysfunction of vasoregulatory control can lead to vasospasm, defined as inappropriate tone of an artery or vein that results in impaired vasodilatation with increased physiologic demand, leading to tissue ischemia manifested as cold intolerance or tissue death. If vasospasm occurs in the setting of underlying occlusive disease, distal ulceration or gangrene can occur within the digits. Vasospastic disease can be classified as either primary or secondary; primary vasospasm exists independently without an identifiable cause,

The authors have nothing to disclose.
[a] Division of Plastic Surgery, University of Pennsylvania Hershey Medical Center, 500 University Drive, Hershey, PA 17033, USA; [b] Department of Orthopedics and Division of Plastic Surgery, Mayo Clinic, 200 First Street Southwest, Rochester, MN 55905, USA
* Corresponding author. Mayo Clinic, 12th Floor, 200 First Street Southwest, Rochester, MN 55905.
E-mail address: Moran.steven@mayo.edu

0749-0712/15/$ – see front matter © 2015 Elsevier Inc. All rights reserved.

whereas secondary vasospasm is the result of an existing disease such as systemic sclerosis.

Vaso-occlusive disease differs from vasospastic disease in that the pathogenic mechanism leading to signs and symptoms associated with ischemia are a result of thrombus formation and the remodeling of the intima of small vessels. Immune-mediated vessel remodeling can result from stimulation or destruction of cells within the vessels at multiple levels, such as the endothelial cell, smooth muscle cell, pericyte, or adventitial fibroblast.[1] Autoantibody formation and deposition along with complement activation may lead to inflammatory changes and vessel fibrosis.[2] Inflammatory thrombi may form in the presence of irritants such as tobacco; in such cases pathologic intravascular changes can result in thrombus formation in the absence of complement activation or disruption of the intima media or adventitia, as seen in Buerger disease.[3] Vaso-occlusive disease can also develop in the setting of repetitive trauma, leading to aneurysm formation, thrombus, and thromboemboli, as seen in cases of hypothenar hammer syndrome. Because vaso-occlusive disease of the hand can be present within a broad spectrum of underlying pathophysiologic conditions, a thorough history and physical examination is imperative in guiding treatment.

SCLERODERMA

The main features of this complex disease, also known as systemic sclerosis, include tissue fibrosis, changes in host vasculature, and the formation of autoantibodies directed at many different host proteins. The estimated prevalence of scleroderma is variable and ranges from 50 to 300 persons per 1 million.[4] There are 2 further classifications for scleroderma: limited cutaneous scleroderma and diffuse cutaneous scleroderma.[5] Limited scleroderma is usually confined to the hands, arms, and face, and often presents as isolated Raynaud phenomenon before development of tissue fibrosis. Also associated with limited cutaneous scleroderma is the presence of pulmonary fibrosis and anticentromere antibodies in up to 90% of patients.[1] Diffuse cutaneous scleroderma, a term often used synonymously with CREST syndrome (Calcinosis, Raynaud phenomenon, Esophageal dysmotility, Sclerodactyly, Telangiectasias), is a progressive disorder that affects a significant amount of skin and, commonly, 1 or more internal organs. Patients may also display features of other autoimmune conditions such as systemic lupus erythematosus (SLE; lupus), Sjögren disease, rheumatoid arthritis, or polymyositis.

Scleroderma can have functionally debilitating consequences in the upper extremity. Changes commonly associated with sclerosis of the hand include Raynaud phenomenon, arthropathy, and calcinosis.[6] Triggered by a cold stimulus or other environmental stressor, Raynaud phenomenon results in blanching, cyanosis, and reactive hyperemia. Raynaud phenomenon is due to unopposed vasoconstriction of the small vessels of the hand (**Fig. 1**). Histopathologic changes affecting the vessels are preceded by immune-mediated vascular injury, which affects essentially all vessels, including those in the hands. Damage is initiated by immune-mediated damage to the endothelium with generation of reactive oxygen species. Early stages of scleroderma are marked by perivascular invasion of mononuclear cells, release of inflammatory cytokines, and activation of smooth muscle cells, resulting in intimal hyperplasia and vasospasm ultimately leading to Raynaud phenomenon. Later stages of vascular disease include migration and activation of fibroblasts in the perivascular space leading to excessive collagen deposition, fibrosis, and rarefaction of capillaries.[7–11]

Raynaud phenomenon can precede other signs of systemic sclerosis by several years. Intimal hyperplasia and later fibrosis of the vessels lead to progressively worsened ischemia distal to the level of disease, with resulting ulceration and gangrenous changes. Common locations for ulceration include the fingertip and over the proximal interphalangeal (PIP) and metacarpophalangeal (MP) joints (**Fig. 2**). Ulceration of the fingertip can be related to both ischemia and calcinosis. Wounds over joints, specifically the PIP joint, can result from flexion contracture and sclerosis of the skin (**Figs. 3** and **4**). Nonhealing wounds over joints can lead to osteomyelitis or septic arthritis.

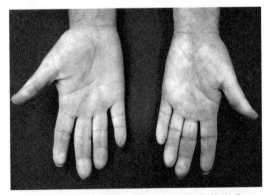

Fig. 1. A 50-year-old woman with limited scleroderma displaying the appearance of Raynaud phenomenon. In addition, one can see evidence of cutaneous involvement throughout the hand.

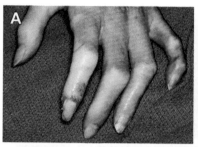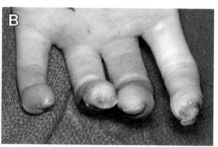

Fig. 2. (*A*) A 56-year-old woman with limited cutaneous scleroderma resulting in severe Raynaud phenomenon of the fingers with associated loss of soft tissue. (*B*) Common locations for ulceration include the fingertip and over the proximal interphalangeal and metacarpophalangeal joints.

Raynaud phenomenon associated with systemic sclerosis is often treated conservatively through avoidance of environmental stressors, smoking cessation, and medical therapy with vasodilation agents. Nonsurgical pharmacotherapy includes calcium-channel blockade, serotonin antagonism, intra-arterial reserpine injection, and subcutaneous injection of botulinum toxin (Botox).[12–15] Surgery may be indicated when conservative treatment has failed or the disease continues to progress. Soft-tissue ulceration can quickly lead to soft-tissue infection and digital loss. In such cases, the authors are aggressive with wound care in addition to medical management and Botox injections. If these therapies fail to improve or halt the loss of soft tissue, the authors recommend surgical intervention to improve blood flow. In most cases sympathectomies can be used to decrease vasoconstriction.

The sympathetic nervous system is responsible for generating the signals leading to vasoconstriction. Because these nerves travel within the adventitia of the peripheral vasculature, surgical adventitial stripping can be performed, reducing

sympathetic vasoconstriction and leading to increased peripheral blood flow.[16] Sympathetic tone can be disrupted at several different levels. Cervicothoracic sympathectomy may be performed to improve distal blood flow by ablation of the cervical sympathetic trunk. Surgical sympathectomy at this level can be approached in transaxillary, supraclavicular, or thoracoscopic manner, whereby resection of the T1 to T4 ganglia is usually performed. Patients often have initial improvement or resolution of their symptoms with healing of digital ulceration; unfortunately, nearly all patients will experience return of symptoms between 6 and 12 months following surgery. High recurrence rates along with the risk of Horner syndrome following this procedure have resulted in a shift toward more distal sympathectomy.[17]

In the presence of vaso-occlusive disease, distal blood flow can be restored by sympathectomy performed concomitantly with ligation of the thrombosed or occluded vascular segment. As originally described by Leriche,[18] a segment of the superficial palmar arch can be resected with resultant removal of the coexisting peri-arterial

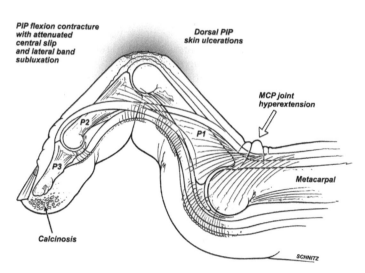

Fig. 3. Scleroderma can lead to soft-tissue fibrosis and proximal interphalangeal (PIP) contracture within the fingers. Over time, stretch of the central slip and fibrosis of the volar plate can result in PIP flexion contractures, ulceration, and bone exposure at the PIP joint. Compensatory hyperextension of metacarpophalangeal (MCP) joint can occur. Calcinosis at the level of the distal phalanx in conjunction with vasculitis contributes to tissue loss. P1, proximal phalanx; P2, middle phalanx; P3, distal phalanx. (*From* Jakubietz MG, Jakubietz RG, Gruenert JG. Scleroderma of the hand. J Am Soc Surg Hand 2005;5(1):42–7; with permission.)

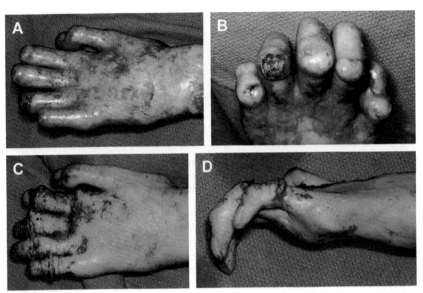

Fig. 4. A 37-year-old man with a history of CREST syndrome with significant involvement of both upper extremities. (*A, B*) Typical hand deformity, as described in **Fig. 3**, with ulceration of proximal interphalangeal (PIP) joints and fixed flexion contractures, making hand use minimal. (*C, D*) Management of the soft tissues and joint is carried out with PIP fusions, which allow for placing PIP joints in a position of function. PIP fusion with tension band technique also corrects compensatory hyperextension of metacarpophalangeal joint and allows for primary closure of dorsal PIP skin with minimal hardware bulk.

sympathetic fibers, with or without subsequent arterial reconstruction, usually performed by interposing a reversed saphenous vein graft. With the advent of microsurgical techniques, it has become possible to disrupt the sympathetic fibers without resection of a segment of an artery.[19] The decision to reconstruct the resected arterial segment is controversial, and there exists no level-1 or level-2 evidence in support of reconstruction. Intraoperative testing can be performed to aid in the decision of whether to reconstructing the artery should include digital-brachial indices (normal >0.7), digital plethysmography, and pulse volume recording, as these diagnostic adjuncts should improve following sympathectomy, with resultant vasodilation. The preoperative and intraoperative assessment may by confounded by the presence of discontinuous occlusive lesions along the length of the digital artery. Ruch and colleagues[20] examined the hands of patients with clinical and arteriographic findings consistent with vaso-occlusive disease of the upper extremity, and found that 25 of 33 hands (76%) had multilevel occlusive disease, of whom 52% had occlusive disease at or distal to the level of the PIP joint. Multilevel disease and distal disease makes it difficult for the surgeon to determine collateral flow with any of the available diagnostic imaging modalities.

Operative Technique for Leriche Sympathectomy

After exsanguination of the affected extremity, tourniquet control is applied and a longitudinal incision is made over the affected segment of artery. Surgical exploration is performed using loupe magnification guided by preoperative arteriography. The patency of the vessel is assessed intraoperatively. The entirety of the thrombosed segment is identified, ligated, and discarded. A dynamic intraoperative assessment of collateral flow should be performed using Doppler, digital plethysmography, or pulse volume recording. If the objective parameters have not improved as a result of the segmental resection, vascular reconstruction can be performed if there are adequate distal target vessels.

Options for arterial reconstruction include reversed vein grafts from the cephalic, basilic or saphenous systems, or arterial grafts using the deep inferior epigastric artery, subscapular artery, thoracodorsal artery, or descending branch of the lateral femoral circumflex artery. Arterial reconstruction with donor arterial graft may have better long-term patency rates. At 18-month follow-up, a meta-analysis by Masden and colleagues[21] demonstrated 100% arterial graft patency versus 85% patency at 37-month follow-up for venous bypass grafts. With arterial reconstruction of the hand there has been improvement in microvascular perfusion, as evidenced by laser Doppler and increase in distal temperature measurements. Hand symptoms and function improve as a result of arterial reconstruction; however, cold sensitivity, as demonstrated by McCabe score, does not improve as a result of arterial reconstruction.[22]

Operative Technique for Periarterial Sympathectomy

The goal of the peripheral or periarterial sympathectomy is to disrupt the sympathetic connections from the peripheral nerves of the hand to the peripheral blood vessels (**Fig. 5**). Techniques to disrupt sympathetic innervation at multiple levels have been described with various modifications in techniques. Flatt[23] originally described the digital sympathectomy, whereby either horizontal or Brunner incisions are performed over the affected digit distal to the common digital neurovascular bundle, allowing wide exposure of the digital neurovascular bundles. Intervening nerve fibers are transected, and a short-segment (3–4 mm) of the adventitia is stripped from the radial and ulnar digital arteries of the affected digits.[23]

Modifications of this technique by Koman and colleagues[24] have led to the development of peripheral sympathectomy of the entire affected hand. Using the principle of disrupting the sympathetic fibers that run within the arterial adventitia, Koman and colleagues[24] designed an operation to surgically excise the adventitia at multiple levels about the hand and wrist. The procedure begins with longitudinal incisions made volar to the radial and ulnar arteries proximal to the distal wrist crease. The arteries are exposed and circumferentially dissected whereby 2 cm of adventitia is removed. The next incision is carried out over the superficial palmar arch at the distal wrist crease. The common digital neurovascular bundles are identified, and connections between the arteries and nerves are transected. Several millimeters of adventitia are stripped from the bifurcation of the common digital artery from the superficial palmar arch. Finally, a fourth dorsal incision is made if the patient has thumb symptoms. This longitudinal incision is carried out over the anatomic snuffbox where the radial artery is identified, and several millimeters of adventitia are removed from the origin of the deep palmar arch.

Ruch and colleagues[25] evaluated the effect of periarterial sympathectomy in 29 hands in patients with scleroderma. Each of these patients had documented systemic sclerosis and chronic vascular insufficiency with nonhealing digital ulcers that were nonresponsive to nonoperative

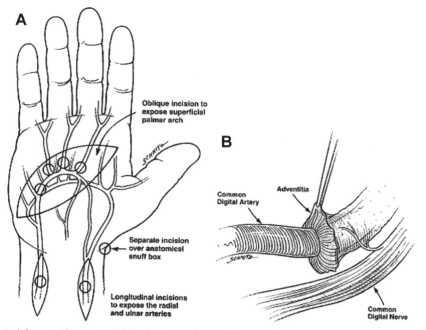

Fig. 5. Periarterial sympathectomy. (A) Typical areas for making incisions when performing a periarterial sympathectomy. (B) Technique of microvascular adventitial stripping of the common digital arteries, which separates the sympathetic fibers that travel with the common digital nerves. (*From* Ruch DS, Koman LA, Smith TL. Chronic vascular disorders of the upper extremity. J Am Soc Surg. Hand 2001;1(1);73–9; with permission.)

treatment. After a mean follow-up of 31 months, patients demonstrated increased microvascular perfusion, as demonstrated by laser Doppler, and subjective improvement in ulcer burden in 86% of patients, but variable improvement in symptom severity. Because of the progressive nature of the disease, 75% of patients in this study did eventually develop additional ulcerations or tissue necrosis despite surgical treatment.

Hartzell and colleagues[26] examined the results of 33 extremities (59 digits) with clinically proven vaso-occlusive disease of either immune-mediated or atherosclerotic etiology. After failing nonsurgical treatment, patients underwent peripheral sympathectomy at the level of the common digital neurovascular bundles. Patients were then evaluated in terms of ulcer healing and amputation based on the cause of their vaso-occlusive disease. After an average follow-up of 96 months, 28 of 42 digits in the immune-mediated vasculitis group had a decrease in ulcer number or went on to heal completely; by comparison, only 2 of 17 digits affected by atherosclerotic disease showed improvement in ulcer number or went on to heal completely. A greater number of patients (10 of 17) in the atherosclerosis group went on to digital amputation, compared with 11 of 42 patients in the immune-mediated vasculitis group. These data suggest that peripheral sympathectomy may provide some benefit in the setting the vaso-occlusive disease related to an autoimmune condition, but has very little benefit in atherosclerotic disease.

Multiple soft-tissue and bony deformities can develop scleroderma in conjunction with vasculitis. Such deformities when combined with hand ischemia can create challenging problems for the hand surgeon (see **Fig. 3**). Indications for bony reconstructive procedures in the management of scleroderma include loss of function and motion, skin at risk, and infection. The most common surgical treatment options include arthrodesis, arthroplasty, and amputation. Because of the generally poor quality of the skin and soft tissues, bony reconstructions tend to be favored over soft-tissue procedures. Providing a tension-free skin closure is an essential premise in optimizing outcomes following surgery, and minimizing the risk of wound healing problems and infection.

PIP fusion is the most common reconstructive procedure for scleroderma. Melone and colleagues[27] reported that interphalangeal (IP) arthrodesis accounted for nearly 80% of 272 procedures performed at their institution. Arthrodesis is preferred by most surgeons over arthroplasty for the IP joints. Norris and Brown noted that range of motion following PIP arthroplasty in patients with scleroderma was only 30° and the implant failure rate was 10%.[28] As many of these patients have significant flexion of the PIP joint, an arthrodesis has the benefit of relieving the tension on the dorsal skin and slightly shortening the digit. An arthroplasty carries the risk of recurrent deformity, which can exacerbate the dorsal skin tension and invite wound problems on the dorsum of the PIP joint.

The technique can be performed with regional anesthesia, and a longitudinal dorsal incision used. Care should be taken to gently raise thick tissue flaps and avoid overly aggressive handling of the skin. The tendon is then split longitudinally to expose the joint. Liberal resection of the joint will help correct the deformity and allow for ideal positioning of the fusion. In addition, if a preexisting dorsal wound exists, the defect can often be debrided and primarily closed. Jones and colleagues[6] reported that a position of 45° to 55° of flexion was functionally satisfactory and allowed for excellent thumb opposition to the digit. Kirschner wires and tension band is an effective way to stabilize the construct, having the advantages of being rigid and with a low profile. The tendon layer is then reapproximated with the distal IP joint flexed to minimize tendency for hyperextension. The skin is closed with nonabsorbable interrupted sutures. Postoperatively, the finger is immobilized until wound healing.

Occasionally the MP joint will require surgical attention, usually in addition to the PIP joint. In contrast to the flexion deformity of the PIP joint, the MP joint is deformed into a hyperextended position. Both resection and silicone implant arthroplasty have been described.[6,27] The technique for the MP joint requires gentle manipulation of the skin, taking care to protect the dorsal interweb space veins. A wide bony resection including complete metacarpal head removal is often necessary. In addition, the collateral ligaments and soft-tissue supporting structures typically need to be released to correct the deformity. Liberal bony shortening of the metacarpal will also allow for a tension-free skin closure. Melone and colleagues[27] preferred the use of arthroplasty, and reported gratifying outcomes with silicone implants up to 15 years after surgery. Jones and colleagues,[6] however, preferred resection arthroplasty.

Calcinosis cutis is commonly seen in patients with scleroderma. Radiographically they can be either focal or diffuse in appearance. Indications for treatment include pain, extrusion through the skin, and functional impairment. Surgically, excision is aimed at effectively debulking the accumulated calcinosis. Overly aggressive resection may devascularize the digits. Mendelson and colleagues[29] reported the use of pulsed irrigation and burr to help break up the calcific mass while debriding. Unfortunately, recurrence is not uncommon.

SYSTEMIC LUPUS ERYTHEMATOSUS

SLE ranges in prevalence from 40 to 200 per 100,000 persons for those who are of Northern Europeans or African descent.[30] Although the life expectancy of SLE has improved dramatically over the last 50 years, 15-year survival rates following diagnosis is still only 80%.[31] The pathophysiology of lupus is not completely understood. Patients develop autoantibodies directed at double-stranded DNA and other non-DNA antigens including Ro (a ribonucleoprotein complex), La (an RNA-binding protein), C1q (a subunit of the C1 complement component), Sm (nuclear particles composed of small polypeptides), and others.[2] These autoantibodies activate complement and initiate an inflammatory response following host cell apoptosis, phagocytosis, and antigen presentation. Although autoantibodies do exist in individuals without causing lupus-type symptoms, patients who eventually develop features of the disease generate autoantibodies with a high affinity for antigen, which leads to increased stimulation of B cells with resultant production of more antibody in the presence of T-cell costimulation in what is known as an antigen-driven response.[2]

Lupus, like scleroderma, may manifest initially as Raynaud phenomenon, and this symptom alone can precede a diagnosis of systemic disease for several years. Other vascular sequelae associated with SLE include peripheral arterial occlusion, chronic lower extremity ulceration, livedo reticularis, and recurrent thrombophlebitis.[32] The etiology of peripheral vascular disease in lupus is multifactorial, and is thought to result from immune-mediated inflammation within the blood vessels in addition to commonly associated comorbid conditions such as insulin resistance, dyslipidemias, and hypertension, which accelerate the development of atherosclerosis.

Upper extremity vascular problems are most commonly seen in patients with evidence of antiphospholipid antibodies. These patients are at risk for antiphospholipid syndrome,[33] which is diagnosed by the presence of antiphospholipid antibodies and signs and symptoms associated with vascular thrombosis, stroke, and venous thromboembolism.[34] Although venous thromboembolic events are encountered more commonly, peripheral arterial thrombosis can also occur. Up to 26.6% of patients with antiphospholipid

syndrome can develop severe upper extremity ischemic complications.[34,35] In a large multicenter study of 637 lupus patients, peripheral vascular disease was diagnosed in 5.3% of the cohort. Of these patients with vascular disease, 19 (55%) were reported to have minor tissue loss and 7 (21%) had significant tissue loss, as denoted by amputation of digit or extremity (foot). None of the patients in this study underwent a revascularization before amputation.[36]

Raynaud phenomenon associated with lupus occurs in 16% to 40% of patients, and should be managed initially with avoidance of triggers and/or disease-modifying medical therapy.[34,37] Medications used to control ischemic pain and cold sensitivity associated with Raynaud phenomenon include vasodilating agents as previously described for patients with scleroderma. If the peripheral vaso-occlusive disease worsens or is associated with distal digital necrosis refractory to medical management, Botox injection or surgical intervention should be considered. Preoperative angiography can aid in the diagnosis and localization of vaso-occlusive lesions. If identified, a thrombosed arterial segment can be removed and a revascularization can be performed using either a vein or arterial graft. Digital or peripheral sympathectomy can be performed, where indicated, for concomitant refractory vasospastic disease.

Multiple soft-tissue and bony deformities can be associated with hand ischemia seen in lupus. The ligament laxity and joint disease associated with SLE results in hand deformities similar to those seen in rheumatoid arthritis. The fingers will typically deviate ulnarly at the MP joints while the PIP joints may develop hyperextension or (to a lesser extent) flexion and angular deformities. For patients who fail conservative treatments and have ongoing pain or dysfunction, surgery is indicated.

MP joint disease and deformity can be managed with extensor tendon centralization and soft-tissue balancing if the joint is passively correctable and the patient has minimal or no joint destruction. In cases with substantial joint disease or fixed contracture, an MP arthroplasty is helpful in both alleviating pain and maintaining the corrected alignment. The MP joints can be approached via individual longitudinal incisions centered over each joint or with a single transverse incision. Care is taken to protect and preserve the dorsal veins. The tendon layer is approached from the radial side to allow for plication for the centralization. The joint capsule can be split longitudinally to reveal the joint. If the joint is preserved, a synovectomy can be performed, and the ligaments can be identified and tightened radially to help correct the deformity, with or without release or lengthening ulnarly. If the joint is replaced, the silicone hinged implants have the advantage of providing inherent stability. The ulnar intrinsics are step-cut lengthened. In some cases complete release or cross-intrinsic transfers has been used to help maintain the correction. However, Dray and colleagues[38] cautioned against complete intrinsic release and transfer in the treatment of SLE. These investigators noted that such procedures, which are typical in the management of rheumatoid arthritis, have resulted in a few fingers of overcorrection in the management of SLE. On closure, the extensor tendon can be tightened (in addition to centralized) to help maintain an extended MP joint position. Some surgeons have proposed and used suturing of the extensor tendon to the central dorsal aspect of the proximal phalanx to help maintain correction.[39] Postoperatively, the patient is placed in a splint maintaining the MP joints in extension for 4 to 6 weeks. The patient then graduates to static splinting with or without dynamic splinting. Static splints are used for nighttime use for 6 to 12 months.

The PIP joints in SLE are most commonly hyperextended with a swan-neck deformity. General treatment principles apply to the treatment of swan-neck deformities. If the joint is passively correctable, procedures such as lateral band relocation, superficialis hemitenodesis, and dorsal capsulotomy can be considered. It is important that the underlying pathology of SLE affects both the intrinsic and extrinsic muscles/tendons. Thus, correction of the deformity needs to address both, and unfortunately can be difficult to maintain. Often fusion is the only practical treatment, especially in cases where the joint develops a fixed deformity. Correction of the PIP joint is often necessary to maintain MP joint realignment over the long term.[38]

BUERGER DISEASE

Buerger disease, also referred to as thromboangiitis obliterans, is a disease that results in segmental vascular inflammation and thrombus formation, and affects small and medium-sized arteries and veins.[40] Histologically this disease entity differs from other forms of autoimmune vasculitis in that the blood-vessel wall is free of inflammatory changes, but within the vessel lumen there are highly cellular inflammatory thrombus. Markers of inflammation, such as C-reactive protein and erythrocyte sedimentation rate, are typically normal in cases of Buerger disease. Immunologic indicators, such as complement, immune complexes, and cryoglobulins, are also often normal; however, the thrombus itself demonstrates features of an immune-mediated process.[41]

The disease affects 12.6 per 100,000 persons in the United States, of whom up to 80% are of Ashkenazi Jewish descent.[40] Although the exact pathogenesis is incompletely understood, tobacco use has been clearly linked with progression of the disease process.[42] As determined by Makita and colleagues,[43] impairment of endothelial-dependent relaxation seems to be centrally related to disease pathogenesis.

The disease is typically classified into acute, intermediate, and chronic, depending on the histologic progression of the thrombus. In the acute phase, a vessel biopsy may reveal a highly cellular, inflammatory thrombus in both the arterial and venous system, with relative preservation of the 3 components of the vessel wall. By contrast, in atherosclerosis and other vasculopathies, the internal elastic lamina and media are typically involved in the disease process.[40]

Clinically, Buerger disease is usually seen in young male smokers, presenting with claudication of the extremities. The disease typically begins with the distal arteries and veins, and may result in rest pain and ischemic ulcerations as it progresses. In a study from Cleveland Clinic, 112 patients with Buerger disease were evaluated from 1970 to 1987, and distal ischemic ulcers were apparent at the time of presentation in 76% of patients.[42] The disease typically involves more than 1 limb; therefore, it may be practical to investigate all limbs during the initial workup.[40] It is prudent to rule out other sources of distal arterial occlusion that may result from underlying connective tissue disorders such as SLE, or systemic sclerosis (CREST syndrome), especially when patients present with Raynaud phenomenon. Traumatic thromboembolic disease (hypothenar hammer syndrome) can mimic Buerger disease and can be effectively excluded with extremity arteriography. A cardiac thrombus with distal emboli-related ischemic changes should also be considered and, if there exists and high index of suspicion, a cardiac ultrasonogram can be performed. Although many different diagnostic criteria exist, Olin[40] propose that Buerger disease should be diagnosed by the presence of the following characteristics: (1) age less than 45 years, (2) prior or current history of tobacco use, (3) distal extremity ischemia confirmed by noninvasive vascular studies, (4) exclusion of confounding comorbidities such as other connective tissue diseases, hypercoagulable state, and diabetes mellitus, and (5) exclusion of a proximal embolic source. "Corkscrew collaterals" may be seen on angiography (**Fig. 6**).

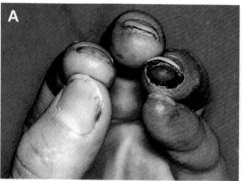 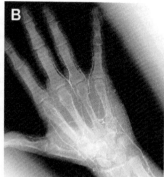

Fig. 6. A 28-year-old man with diagnosis of Buerger disease. (*A*) The patient's fingers show evidence of ongoing ischemia and distal tip necrosis in addition to splinter hemorrhages in nail beds, indicating underlying embolic disease. (*B*) Angiogram shows minimal flow to fingers and evidence of early "corkscrew collaterals" at the level of the common digital arteries, and significant collaterals through the hypothenar musculature.

Treatment of Buerger disease is primarily nonsurgical and begins with complete cessation of all tobacco products.[44] Olin reports a series of 120 patients with Buerger disease in which 94% of patients who successfully abstained from tobacco products avoided amputation. By contrast, 43% of patients who continued smoking required amputations.[3] Patients may continue to have Raynaud phenomenon despite cessation of smoking, and therefore may benefit from peripheral sympathectomy and surgical revascularization in the setting of occlusive thrombosis.

Buerger disease is often segmental in nature, with several areas of distal thrombosis increasing the difficulty of surgical revascularization because of the absence of a suitable recipient artery distal to the level of occlusion. If progressive ischemia exists in the patient for whom an arteriogram suggests the presence of an adequate recipient artery, autologous venous or arterial grafting should be attempted. Patients who continue to smoke following bypass grafting have a lower rate of graft patency than those who discontinue smoking (35% patent in smokers vs 67% patent in nonsmokers).[45] A surgical alternative to revascularization alone is the transfer of an omental free flap. Singh and Ramteke[46] reported a series of 50 patients who underwent omental transfer for Buerger disease whereby 72% of patients had decreased pain at rest and 88% of patients in whom ulcers were present had healed their ulcers following surgery.

SUMMARY

Vasospastic symptoms are common with scleroderma, lupus, and Buerger disease. Fortunately medical therapy is effective in managing symptoms in many of these individuals. Recent success

with Botox injections has provided new hope for patients wishing to avoid surgery. The authors have found a positive response to Botox to be predictive of surgical success with distal sympathectomies, should surgery be necessary in certain cases. If patients fail medical management, distal sympathectomies in conjunction with vascular reconstruction can help in preventing tissue loss and preserving hand function.

REFERENCES

1. Gabrielli A, Avvedimento EV, Krieg T. Scleroderma. N Engl J Med 2009;360(19):1989–2003.
2. Rahman A, Isenberg DA. Systemic lupus erythematosus. N Engl J Med 2008;358(9):929–39.
3. Olin JW. Thromboangiitis obliterans (Buerger's disease). N Engl J Med 2000;343(12):864–9.
4. Chifflot H, Fautrel B, Sordet C, et al. Incidence and prevalence of systemic sclerosis: a systematic literature review. Semin Arthritis Rheum 2008;37(4):223–35.
5. LeRoy EC, Black C, Fleischmajer R, et al. Scleroderma (systemic sclerosis): classification, subsets and pathogenesis. J Rheumatol 1988;15(2):202–5.
6. Jones NF, Imbriglia JE, Steen VD, et al. Surgery for scleroderma of the hand. J Hand Surg 1987;12(3): 391–400.
7. Kahaleh B. Vascular disease in scleroderma: mechanisms of vascular injury. Rheum Dis Clin North Am 2008;34(1):57–71, vi.
8. Kraling BM, Maul GG, Jimenez SA. Mononuclear cellular infiltrates in clinically involved skin from patients with systemic sclerosis of recent onset predominantly consist of monocytes/macrophages. Pathobiology 1995;63(1):48–56.
9. Rajkumar VS, Sundberg C, Abraham DJ, et al. Activation of microvascular pericytes in autoimmune Raynaud's phenomenon and systemic sclerosis. Arthritis Rheum 1999;42(5):930–41.

10. LeRoy EC. Increased collagen synthesis by sclero-derma skin fibroblasts in vitro: a possible defect in the regulation or activation of the scleroderma fibro-blast. J Clin Invest 1974;54(4):880–9.

11. Eckes B, Mauch C, Hüppe G, et al. Differential regulation of transcription and transcript stability of pro-alpha 1(I) collagen and fibronectin in activated fibroblasts derived from patients with systemic scleroderma. Biochem J 1996;315(Pt 2):549–54.

12. Rademaker M, Cooke ED, Almond NE, et al. Comparison of intravenous infusions of iloprost and oral nifedipine in treatment of Raynaud's phenomenon in patients with systemic sclerosis: a double blind randomised study. BMJ 1989;298(6673):561–4.

13. Seibold JR, Jageneau AH. Treatment of Raynaud's phenomenon with ketanserin, a selective antagonist of the serotonin2 (5-HT2) receptor. Arthritis Rheum 1984;27(2):139–46.

14. Hurst LN, Evans HB, Brown DH. Vasospasm control by intra-arterial reserpine. Plast Reconstr Surg 1982; 70(5):595–9.

15. Neumeister MW. Botulinum toxin type A in the treatment of Raynaud's phenomenon. J Hand Surg 2010; 35(12):2085–92.

16. Barcroft H, Walker AJ. Return to tone in blood-vessels of the upper limb after sympathectomy. Lancet 1949;1(6564):1035–9.

17. Lowell RC, Gloviczki P, Cherry KJ Jr, et al. Cervico-thoracic sympathectomy for Raynaud's syndrome. Int Angiol 1993;12(2):168–72.

18. Leriche R. Treatment of pain by sympathectomy. Rev Neurol (Paris) 1950;83(1):41–2.

19. Kleinert HE, Volianitis GJ. Thrombosis of the palmar arterial arch and its tributaries: etiology and newer concepts in treatment. J Trauma 1965;5:447–57.

20. Ruch DS, Smith TL, Smith BP, et al. Anatomic and physiologic evaluation of upper extremity ischemia. Microsurgery 1999;19(4):181–8.

21. Masden DL, Seruya M, Higgins JP. A systematic review of the outcomes of distal upper extremity bypass surgery with arterial and venous conduits. J Hand Surg 2012;37(11):2362–7.

22. Ruch DS, Aldridge M, Holden M, et al. Arterial reconstruction for radial artery occlusion. J Hand Surg 2000;25(2):282–90.

23. Flatt AE. Digital artery sympathectomy. J Hand Surg 1980;5(6):550–6.

24. Koman LA, Smith BP, Pollock FE Jr, et al. The micro-circulatory effects of peripheral sympathectomy. J Hand Surg 1995;20(5):709–17.

25. Ruch DS, Holden M, Smith BP, et al. Periarterial sympathectomy in scleroderma patients: intermediate-term follow-up. J Hand Surg 2002;27(2):258–64.

26. Hartzell TL, Makhni EC, Sampson C. Long-term results of periarterial sympathectomy. J Hand Surg 2009;34(8):1454–60.

27. Melone CP, McLoughlin JC, Beldner S. Surgical management of the hand in scleroderma. Curr Opin Rheumatol 1999;11(6):514–20.

28. Norris RW, Brown HG. The proximal interphalangeal joint in systemic sclerosis and its surgical management. Br J Plast Surg 1985;38(4):526–31.

29. Mendelson BC, Linscheid RL, Dobyns JH, et al. Surgical treatment of calcinosis cutis in the upper extremity. J Hand Surg Am 1977;2(4):318–24.

30. Johnson AE, Gordon C, Palmer RG, et al. The prevalence and incidence of systemic lupus erythe-matosus in Birmingham, England. Relationship to ethnicity and country of birth. Arthritis Rheum 1995;38(4):551–8.

31. Abu-Shakra M, Urowitz MB, Gladman DD, et al. Mortality studies in systemic lupus erythematosus. Results from a single center. I. Causes of death. J Rheumatol 1995;22(7):1259–64.

32. Alarcon Segovia D, Osmundson PJ. Peripheral vascular syndromes associated with systemic lupus erythematosus. Ann Intern Med 1965;62:907–19.

33. Kao AH, Sabatine JM, Manzi S. Update on vascular disease in systemic lupus erythematosus. Curr Opin Rheumatol 2003;15(5):519–27.

34. Cervera R, Boffa MC, Khamashta MA, et al. The Euro-Phospholipid project: epidemiology of the anti-phospholipid syndrome in Europe. Lupus 2009; 18(10):889–93.

35. Asherson RA, Cervera R, Shoenfeld Y. Peripheral vascular occlusions leading to gangrene and ampu-tations in antiphospholipid antibody positive patients. Ann N Y Acad Sci 2007;1108:515–29.

36. Burgos PI, Vilá LM, Reveille JD, et al. Peripheral vascular damage in systemic lupus erythematosus: data from LUMINA, a large multi-ethnic U.S. cohort (LXIX). Lupus 2009;18(14):1303–8.

37. Greco CM, Rudy TE, Manzi S. Adaptation to chronic pain in systemic lupus erythematosus: applicability of the multidimensional pain inventory. Pain Med 2003;4(1):39–50.

38. Dray GJ, Millender LH, Nalebuff EA, et al. The surgical treatment of hand deformities in systemic lupus erythematosus. J Hand Surg Am 1981;6(4): 339–45.

39. Wood VE, Ichtertz DR, Yahiku H. Soft tissue meta-carpophalangeal reconstruction for treatment of rheumatoid hand deformity. J Hand Surg Am 1989; 14(2 Pt 1):163–74.

40. Olin JW. Thromboangiitis obliterans. Curr Opin Rheumatol 1994;6(1):44–9.

41. Kobayashi M, Ito M, Nakagawa A, et al. Immunohis-tochemical analysis of arterial wall cellular infiltration in Buerger's disease (endarteritis obliterans). J Vasc Surg 1999;29(3):451–8.

42. Olin JW, Young JR, Graor RA, et al. The changing clinical spectrum of thromboangiitis obliterans

(Buerger's disease). Circulation 1990;82(5 Suppl): IV3–8.

43. Makita S, Nakamura M, Murakami H, et al. Impaired endothelium-dependent vasorelaxation in peripheral vasculature of patients with thromboangiitis obliterans (Buerger's disease). Circulation 1996;94(Suppl 9):II211–5.

44. Hooten WM, Bruns HK, Hays JT. Inpatient treatment of severe nicotine dependence in a patient with thromboangiitis obliterans (Buerger's disease). Mayo Clin Proc 1998;73(6):529–32.

45. Sasajima T, Kubo Y, Inaba M, et al. Role of infrainguinal bypass in Buerger's disease: an eighteen-year experience. Eur J Vasc Endovasc Surg 1997;13(2): 186–92.

46. Singh I, Ramteke VK. The role of omental transfer in Buerger's disease: New Delhi's experience. Aust N Z J Surg 1996;66(6):372–6.

Revascularization Options for Terminal Distal Ischemia

William C. Pederson, MD

KEYWORDS

- Hand • Ischemia • Bypass • In situ • Venous arterialization • Omental transfer

KEY POINTS

- Direct arterial bypass remains the best option in patients with terminal ischemia of the hand if there is an adequate distal target vessel.
- In situ bypass is the procedure of choice in patients who are candidates for arterial bypass.
- Venous arterialization offers an option in patients in whom there is not adequate arterial runoff in the hand.
- Venous arterialization should be avoided in patients with significant wounds and/or active infection.
- In selected patients, microvascular omental transfer can offer an option for revascularization of the ischemic hand.

INTRODUCTION

Revascularization of the distal hand and fingers remains problematic, because patients with severe vascular disease often lack good outflow in terms of the palmar arch and digital vessels, which may preclude successful arterial-arterial bypass grafting. Many of these patients suffer from severe systemic disease and lower limb loss as well, which can mitigate against complex reconstructive surgery in the upper extremity. These patients especially, however, need their arms and hands, and thus, attempts should be made to salvage the hands whenever possible.

CAUSE

Most patients who suffer from digital ischemia today have a history of collagen vascular disease or diabetes, particularly those diabetics with renal failure. Studies have shown that 17% to 27% of patients with scleroderma will have digital ulcerations requiring some type of treatment.[1] Most of

these will show at least digital artery occlusion, and many will have ulnar artery occlusion on vascular studies.[2] Young diabetics with renal failure are at risk for critical hand ischemia,[3] and those on dialysis are at even higher risk.[3] These patients suffer from calcific vascular disease involving the major vessels and digital vessels in the upper extremity, and the presence of an arteriovenous fistula in the more proximal arm can lead to significant "steal" from the already compromised native circulation. The presence of digital arterial occlusion in both of these groups of patients makes management of their ischemia challenging.

WORKUP

When presented with a patient with impending tissue loss in the hand due to vascular disease, a thorough workup should be done. Most of these patients will already have a known list of medical problems and at least a general internist, endocrinologist, and possibly a nephrologist taking care of

The author has nothing to disclose.
The Hand Center of San Antonio, University of Texas Health Science Center at San Antonio, 21 Spurs Lane, Suite 310, San Antonio, TX 78240, USA
E-mail address: micro1@ix.netcom.com

Hand Clin 31 (2015) 75–83
http://dx.doi.org/10.1016/j.hcl.2014.09.007
0749-0712/15/$ – see front matter © 2015 Elsevier Inc. All rights reserved.

them. They are likely to have already seen a general vascular surgeon, who may have already performed an arteriogram. When the author sees such a patient in the office, he examines them closely to determine the presence of pulses and whether they have had other surgeries (either vascular access procedures or attempts at improving flow). The author performs a "dynamic" Doppler examination on every patient, which involves listening to the radial and ulnar arteries and the palmar arch with alternating occlusion of the radial and ulnar arteries at the wrist. This Doppler examination can usually diagnose distal occlusion of the radial or ulnar artery. The author also listens to each digital pulp to ascertain flow in the digital arteries. In his experience, a vessel at the wrist without a palpable pulse but with a Doppler signal does not mean that there is adequate flow to the hand via this vessel.

The best option remains an arteriogram in evaluating patients with severe ischemia of the hand. The author uses CT angiography (CTA) frequently in patients *without* systemic vascular disease (ulnar or radial artery thrombosis), but the fine detail necessary to evaluate the arch and digital vessels remains lacking in CTA. The author has not found MR angiography to have the level of detail necessary for his purposes. Whether the arteriogram is done by a radiologist or vascular surgeon, it is essential that the hand surgeon views the studies personally to evaluate the vascular system in the forearm and the hand accurately. The author will redo the study if he cannot get a copy of the original arteriogram so that he can evaluate it himself. The decision of what type of surgical intervention to do is usually predicated on the findings on the arteriogram, and thus, the operating surgeon must review the studies himself. Evaluation of the arteriogram is discussed further in the later sections.

NONSURGICAL INTERVENTION

Medical management of patients with critical ischemia of the hand mainly revolves around avoidance of injury to the fingers and hands to prevent ulceration. Patients with diabetes may need to use a site other than the fingertip (such as the earlobe) for checking blood glucose levels to prevent the onset of digital gangrene.[4] Local care of a finger wound once established follows the usual parameters of wound care. In the author's experience with this group of patients, pharmaceutical management with calcium channel blockers and anticoagulants is usually not helpful.

The advent of endovascular surgical procedures has largely changed the management of many

lesions of the lower extremity arterial system. The use of balloon angioplasty and stents has been somewhat limited in the upper extremity, but these techniques are seeing wider application. In a study from Italy, 28 patients underwent angioplasty of diseased arteries below the elbow. Most of these patients suffered from diabetes and were undergoing renal dialysis, and the vessels treated were in the proximal to mid-forearm. These procedures were deemed technically "successful" in 82% of patients, but the hand ulcerations healed in only 65%. In the 18% that were unsuccessful, the vessels were so calcified that the angioplasty catheter could not be passed. In addition, 18% required repeat angioplasty in the first 6 months with some improvement. As would be expected in this severely ill group of patients, more than one-third died during an average of 13 months of follow-up.[5]

More distal use of this technique (at the level of the wrist) has only been reported a few times[6,7] with reasonable short-term success. The author's personal experience with patients managed by the radiologists with angioplasty in the distal forearm has not been good. He has treated several patients after unsuccessful angioplasty who clinically became worse after the attempt, probably because of further compromise of blood flow from a now completely occluded vessel.

SURGICAL MANAGEMENT

The primary options in patients with critical ischemia of the hand are surgical, with direct arterialization still the procedure of choice. Although there have been a few reports of improvement in digital ulcerations in patients with calcific vascular disease after periarterial sympathectomy,[8] the author's results with this technique in this group of patients have been poor. Sympathectomy should be reserved for patients with vasospastic problems, for which this procedure is quite helpful.

If direct arterialization of the arterial system is not an option (due to lack of outflow), then the hand can sometimes be revascularized by other techniques, as discussed below.

DIRECT REVASCULARIZATION

The decision to attempt direct revascularization of the hand is made based on the arteriogram. If there is adequate outflow seen, then direct artery-to-artery bypass via a vein graft is without question the best option. The obvious question is what constitutes adequate outflow and can be a bit difficult to determine if there is high-grade occlusion of the proximal vasculature and very little dye can get into the distal vessels. In the past, the author explored a several of these patients and found, unfortunately, that if there is a proximal high-grade occlusion due to chronic vascular disease, that the distal vessels (radial and/or ulnar arteries) were usually occluded as well. Thus, the decision is based on what distal vessel to target for outflow based on what is visible on the arteriogram. Some cases are fairly straightforward, as in **Fig. 1**, where the arteriogram shows multilevel high-grade stenoses, but with a very reasonable arch and reasonable flow via the digital vessels (see **Fig. 1**). On the other hand, **Fig. 2** shows a much worse situation, but there is some of the deep arch is preserved with some flow to the thumb, index, middle, and little fingers (see **Fig. 2**). Both of these patients would be suitable for in situ vein bypass from the brachial to the radial artery.

The other primary issue in these patients is whether there will be a suitable vein for bypass. The author prefers the "in situ" technique in the arm because the vein wall is thinner than the saphenous (and thus less of a problem to anastomose to the small calcified vessels in the hand) and, if the vein is left in place, the largest part is proximal (for anastomosis to the brachial) and the smallest part is distal. These patients will often have had cardiac revascularization procedures and/or lower extremity revascularizations, which also obviate the use of the saphenous. It is also not uncommon for patients with end-stage vascular disease of the hand to be missing one or both lower extremities.

It may be necessary to explore the arm first to see if either the cephalic or the basilic vein is of adequate diameter and not previously thrombosed from an intravenous line or damaged from

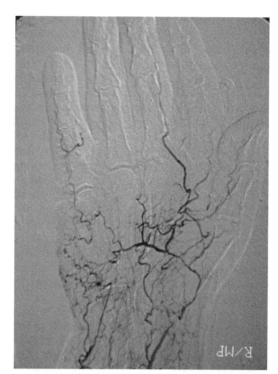

Fig. 2. Arteriogram showing severe blockage in the forearm and only a small amount of the deep arch present, but with digital vessels patent to all of the fingers except the ring finger.

prior arteriovenous fistulae. In most of these patients, the radial artery in the snuffbox is often the best target vessel to restore flow to the arch, and thus, the cephalic vein in the arm is the vein of choice for in situ bypass to this vessel. It is reasonably common to find areas of the cephalic that are occluded, and if these cannot be repaired with another segment of vein, the bypass cannot be performed with the cephalic. The other issue is whether a section of vessel distally can be found that is not so severely calcified that it can be sutured with appropriate-sized suture material for anastomosis of a small artery. The radial artery bifurcates deep within the first web space into the deep palmar arch and the princeps pollicis arteries; often just proximal to the site of this branching there is a small segment of the artery that is soft enough to anastomose to the distal vein using conventional suturing techniques. If the arm veins are inadequate and no leg vein is available, then bypass may not be possible. Likewise, if there is no distal target, vessel bypass may not be an option.

Assuming that the cephalic vein is adequate and that the radial artery in the snuffbox is patent, one can proceed with the bypass. The vein is isolated

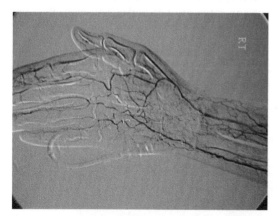

Fig. 1. Arteriogram of a patient with critical ischemia of the hand. Note multiple levels of high-grade stenoses in the radial and ulnar vessels in the distal forearm, but a patent arch and digital vessels going to all fingers.

in its entire length from the antecubital fossa to the wrist. Small branches are all ligated and, if larger branches are present, a few are left temporarily to allow passage of the valvulotome. This vein is then filled with saline and the valvulotome is passed. The author prefers the retrograde Leather Mills type of metal valvulotome, which is passed from distal to proximal and gently pulled through the valves to render them incompetent (**Fig. 3**). The valves in the arm veins are bileaflet, and thus, both leaflets of the valve must be cut with the instrument, or turbulent flow and thrombosis can result. Likewise, valves are often located near branches, and the valvulotome can slice the site of bifurcation of a branch open longitudinally, which presents a difficult injury to repair. Great care must be taken in using the valvulotome in the arm veins because they are thin and can be injured fairly easily. The instrument is generally not long enough to pass all the way up the forearm, and the larger side branches in the mid-forearm can be used to get the more proximal valves. Once the valvulotome has been passed through the length of the vein, the vein is irrigated in an antegrade fashion with heparinized saline to make sure that all of the valves are cut. Once the vein allows for retrograde flow, the proximal anastomosis is performed. The author prefers to do an end-to-side anastomosis between the proximal cephalic vein and the brachial artery in the antecubital fossa. This large anastomosis allows plenty of flow down the vein graft, and the author performs this with a running 6-0 vascular polypropylene. After good flow down the graft is confirmed, the author performs the distal anastomosis at the level of the palm or snuffbox (**Fig. 4**).

In general, this procedure can provide improved blood flow and mitigation of ischemic symptoms and healing of ulcers.[9] Although there are not many large series, 3- to 5-year patency rates are generally reported to be in the range of greater than 80%,[10–12] which mirrors the author's experience with this technique. The author has several patients who have survived their disease for more than 5 years with intact in situ bypass grafts (**Fig. 5**). Although other options exist for the management of patients with end-stage ischemia of the hand, direct arterialization offers the best option if the parameters of available vein and open distal artery for outflow are present.

ARTERIALIZATION OF THE VENOUS SYSTEM

In patients with poor to no outflow vessels available, oxygenated blood can be provided by directing arterial blood flow distally via the intact venous system; this allows arterialized blood to enter the capillary bed in a retrograde fashion. The larger veins require removal of or rendering the valves incompetent to allow for retrograde flow. The smaller veins also contain valves, but these vessels are too small to remove the valves without potentially damaging the vessel. Experimental work has shown that these thin small veins distend when placed under arterial pressure (due to Laplace's law), and this renders the smaller valves incompetent without the need to remove them.[13] Likewise, studies in animals have demonstrated that perfusion via the venous system does provide oxygenated perfusion of the tissues[14,15] and evidence exists that this may lead to angiogenesis in the tissue perfused via the venous system.[16]

Arterialization of the venous system was first used in the lower extremity in cases of poor outflow and would often be combined with arterial bypass (by leaving a branch vein open to allow retrograde perfusion).[17] This technique has shown ongoing promise in patients with few other options and who are at risk for limb loss, and although limb salvage rates are not particularly high, they are

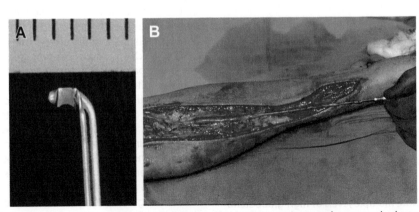

Fig. 3. (*A*) End of Leather Mills retrograde valvulotome. This instrument is passed retrograde down the vein and then gently pulled back to cut the valves. (*B*) Valvulotome being pulled from proximal to distal to cut valves.

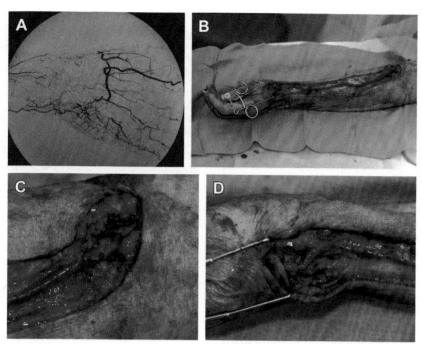

Fig. 4. (*A*) Arteriogram of patient with severe ischemia of the hand and blocked radial and ulnar arteries with reasonable outflow via arch remnant. (*B*) View of arm after bypass from brachial to radial artery with in situ vein. (*C*) View of proximal anastomosis. (*D*) View of distal anastomosis.

usually equal to that of arterial-arterial bypass with poor outflow.[18,19]

This technique was first shown to be efficacious in the upper extremity by King and colleagues[20] in 1993. They performed arterialization of the venous system in 6 limbs of 5 patients and had successful limb salvage in all of them. Other more recent reports have confirmed the efficacy of this approach in patients without other good options for revascularization. Although all of the reported case series are rather small, they all confirm that this technique can lead to decreased pain and healing of ulcers in

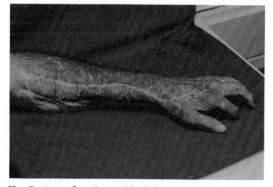

Fig. 5. Arm of patient with diabetes and renal failure 8 years after in situ bypass with no recurrent ulceration or pain.

the chronically ischemic hand.[21–23] Chloros and Koman[24] reported one case with ongoing alleviation of hand symptoms 7 years after arterialization of the venous system.

The author's personal experience with this technique has been reasonable. He has performed arterialization of the venous system in 10 hands in 9 patients. Because of the nature of the underlying disease (usually diabetes and renal failure in the patient population), longevity of this group of patients is not good, and thus, some have been lost to follow-up. Based on patients with good follow-up, there is a moderate early thrombosis rate of around 20% (in the first 6–12 weeks) probably related to ongoing poor outflow and possibly to poor quality of the vein graft used. Of these 2 hands, there was no palpable pulse, but there was still a Doppler signal that could be heard to the level of the metacarpophalangeal joints. Both of these patients did have improvement in pain and ulcerations. One patient suffered an unfortunate thrombosis of a patent venous arterialization bypass when an intravenous line was started in the bypass, despite the protests of the patient. He went on to require vascularized omental transfer. Two other patients lost the operated hand early because of advancing infection. Active infection and large open wounds are the 2 significant contraindications. The author performed venous arterialization in 2 individuals with a wound and mild cellulitis, thinking that improved inflow would help improve the cellulitis (which is often the case with arterial-arterial bypass). Both of these patients required amputation of the hand because of significant increase in the cellulitis and marked swelling in the days after the bypass was performed, despite ongoing antibiotic management and elevation.

The author's technique for venous arterialization is much like the technique of in situ arterial bypass.[25] If there is a major artery (radial or ulnar) open in the forearm, it can be used as proximal inflow for the bypass to an open vein, but these vessels are usually heavily calcified and difficult technically to perform an anastomosis to. The author prefers in most cases to use the cephalic or basilic vein as for an "in situ" type of bypass from the brachial artery to the dorsal hand. The venous system must be examined to see which gives the best flow to the dorsal hand, and ideally that proximal vessel is chosen for anastomosis. Branches in the forearm should be ligated to direct flow into the hand, and the valves in the forearm segment of the vein graft must be removed with a valvulotome as noted above. The author's experience and experimental work have shown that the valves beyond the level of the wrist will become incompetent in the face of arterial pressure. There is no distal anastomosis performed, and blood is allowed to flow retrograde down the forearm "in situ" vein into the dorsal venous system. If there is not good flow to the entire dorsal hand seen after establishing flow via the veins, it can be beneficial to perform an anastomosis between a vein from the side of the hand away from the bypass into the arterialized segment to provide flow to the entire dorsal hand. One can usually detect a Doppler arterial signal to the level of the proximal phalanges in the dorsal veins immediately after this procedure. By several months postoperatively, this signal will usually be found at the level of the dorsal proximal interphalangeal joint (**Fig. 6**).

As noted above, results from this technique can be very good, but they are inferior to arterial-arterial bypass if there is a target artery in the hand that can provide adequate outflow. For venous arterialization to be successful, however, there also has to be an adequate venous system on the dorsal hand and the patient has to be free of infection in the involved extremity (**Fig. 7**).

VASCULARIZED OMENTAL TRANSFER

The potential for management of an extremity with distal ischemia and a wound with combined bypass and soft tissue transfer has been

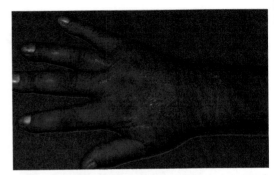

Fig. 6. Hand of patient 6 months after venous arterialization. Marks on dorsal fingers indicate distal extent of arterial Doppler signal in venous system.

discussed for some time.[26] Many articles have been published that showed the utility of this approach, particularly in the lower extremity in the face of poor outflow.[27,28] The addition of a free flap to the bypass certainly improves outflow for the flap and may well provide some element of revascularization of the extremity via angiogenesis from the flap to the limb.[29]

Omentum has long been appreciated to produce angiogenic factors that can be beneficial to healing.[30,31] The omentum has been found to improve wound healing and perfusion in Buerger disease in the lower extremity[32]; this has been applied as a pedicled flap from the abdomen with the omentum stretched out into the leg[33,34] as well as a free flap in some instances.[35] This tissue has also been applied to the upper extremity as a pedicled flap (with later division of the pedicle) with surprisingly good results.[36] It would appear that omental tissue has better ability to revascularize ischemic tissue than a standard fasciocutaneous or muscle flap.

The author has found the omentum to be very effective for revascularization of the upper extremity if no other option exists and when it is reasonable to perform an intra-abdominal procedure on

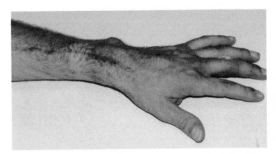

Fig. 7. Patient 3 months after venous arterialization. There is a nearly completely healed eschar over the dorsal ring finger.

the patient. The omentum has been harvested laparoscopically for use as a pedicle flap[37] or as a free flap.[38] Although this would certainly mitigate some of the issues with opening the abdomen, the author has no experience with this approach. Nonetheless, he has performed omental transfer for end-state ischemia of the arm in patients with minimal perioperative morbidity and has had good results in terms of healing of wounds and reversal of ischemic symptoms in these patients. No patients have suffered from intra-abdominal complications, and all patients have healed their wounds. As noted above, this procedure does nothing to change the patient's underlying pathologic condition, and nearly all patients expired within 3 to 5 years of omental transfer because of complications of systemic illness (usually diabetes, renal failure, or posttransplantation issues). Seemingly, this would offer good palliation, however, if the procedure can salvage the upper extremity and improve the patient's quality of life without producing major perioperative morbidity.

Patients who are a candidate for this procedure should have failed standard bypass procedures and/or venous arterializations or not be a candidate for the reasons mentioned above. Likewise, they should be in good enough systemic shape to undergo a general anesthetic as well as an intra-abdominal procedure. The author performs a preoperative vascular study to evaluate where to anastomose the vessels of the omentum, which is usually at the level of the antecubital fossa. The arm is readied for placement of the omentum before harvest. The vessels at the antecubital fossa should be dissected out and readied for anastomosis first. Once this is done, the skin on the dorsum of the volar and dorsal surface of the forearm is incised in small areas, and the skin is elevated off the fascia to allow pockets in which to place the harvested omentum. If the omentum is very bulky and does not fit in the pockets, it may simply be placed on the exposed fascia and covered with a split-thickness skin graft.

The harvest is performed with the assistance of a general surgeon; however the author will dissect the omental vasculature. Based on how much is needed and how large the patient's omentum is, the author may only harvest a portion of the omentum. Knowledge of the vascular anatomy of the omentum is very helpful in this regard, and this should be studied before attempting harvest of the omentum.[39] The omentum is usually harvested on the gastroepiploic and gastoduodenal vessels, which are generally in the 2- to 3-mm range in diameter. Once the harvest is completed, the general surgeon is responsible for closure of the abdomen. The omentum is then placed down the arm on the exposed fascia and in the pockets. Ideally, it will reach the hand but cannot be placed on the palmar surface because of the adherence of the skin to the palmar fascia. If the omentum will not reach the hand, it can simply be placed down to the wrist level. The anastomoses are performed in the proximal forearm, and once this is done, the incisions are closed or the omentum is covered with split-thickness skin graft. If there is a distal target vessel, it is possible to anastomose the distal end of the gastroepiploic artery to this vessel as a flow-through flap.[40] These patients are managed as a standard free flap transfer in terms of postoperative care, but usually these patients will be best managed in the intensive care unit for several days because of their systemic medical issues. The skin grafts will usually have healed by 3 weeks, but improvement in ulcers and rest pain may take 6 to 12 weeks. Surprisingly, some patients who have no Doppler signal in the distal wrist will eventually have return of a biphasic signal in these vessels several months after vascularized omental transfer (**Fig. 8**).

As noted above, results are generally good with this technique and one can expect healing of

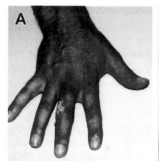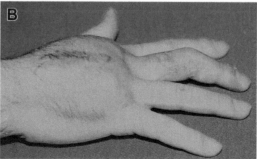

Fig. 8. (*A*) Patient after thrombosis of venous arterialization with worsening ulcer on middle finger. (*B*) Same patient 4 months after vascularized omental transfer to arm and hand. Note dorsal hand mass, which is omentum and healing of ulcer. This patient had return of Doppler arterial signal in the radial artery after 6 months.

ulcers and alleviation of rest pain in most pa-tients.[25,41] Complication rates are fairly low if patient selection is appropriate, but morbidity in the near term remains significant because of the underlying cause of the vascular disease.

REFERENCES

1. Nihtyanova SI, Brough GM, Black CM, et al. Clinical burden of digital vasculopathy in limited and diffuse cutaneous systemic sclerosis. Ann Rheum Dis 2008; 67(1):120–3.
2. Hasegawa M, Nagai Y, Tamura A, et al. Arterio-graphic evaluation of vascular changes of the extremities in patients with systemic sclerosis. Br J Dermatol 2006;155(6):1159–64.
3. Hurton S, Embil JM, Reda A, et al. Upper extremity complications in patients with chronic renal failure receiving haemodialysis. J Ren Care 2010;36(4): 203–11.
4. Dahiya S, Voisine M, Samat A. Gangrene from finger pricking. Endocrine 2012;42(3):767.
5. Ferraresi R, Palloshi A, Aprigliano G, et al. Angio-plasty of below-the-elbow arteries in critical hand ischaemia. Eur J Vasc Endovasc Surg 2012;43(1): 73–80.
6. Namdari S, Park MJ, Weiss AP, et al. Chronic hand ischemia treated with radial artery balloon angio-plasty: case report. J Hand Surg Am 2008;33(4): 551–4.
7. Tasal A, Bacaksiz A, Erdogan E, et al. Successful angioplasty for radial artery chronic total occlusion in a patient with digital gangrene. Postepy Kardiol Interwencyjnej 2013;9(3):304–6.
8. Murata K, Omokawa S, Kobata Y, et al. Long-term follow-up of periarterial sympathectomy for chronic digital ischaemia. J Hand Surg Eur Vol 2012;37(8): 788–93.
9. Cooney WP. Palmar bypass for digital ischemia. J Hand Surg Am 2008;33(4):616–7.
10. Hughes K, Hamdan A, Schermerhorn M, et al. Bypass for chronic ischemia of the upper extremity: results in 20 patients. J Vasc Surg 2007;46(2):303–7.
11. Warren JA, Agarwal G, Wynn JJ. Arterial revascu-larization for upper extremity ischemia in patients with chronic kidney disease. Am Surg 2009; 75(9):848–52.
12. Spinelli F, Benedetto F, Passari G, et al. Bypass surgery for the treatment of upper limb chronic ischaemia. Eur J Vasc Endovasc Surg 2010;39(2): 165–70.
13. Koyama T, Sugihara-Seki M, Sasajima T, et al. Venular valves and retrograde perfusion. Adv Exp Med Biol 2014;812:317–23. http://dx.doi.org/10.1007/978-1-4939-0620-8_42.
14. Koyama T, Sasajima T. Sufficient oxygen can be transported to resting skeletal muscle via arterialization of the vein: theoretical considerations in a rat model. Adv Exp Med Biol 2011;701:335–9.
15. Nichter LS, Haines PC. Arterialized venous perfusion of composite tissue. Am J Surg 1985;150(2):191–6.
16. Sasajima T, Koyama T. Biological maintenance of distal vein arterialization. Adv Exp Med Biol 2013; 765:245–50. http://dx.doi.org/10.1007/978-1-4614-4989-8_34.
17. Sheil GR. Treatment of critical ischaemia of the lower limb by venous arterialization: an interim report. Br J Surg 1977;64(3):197–9.
18. Djoric P. Early individual experience with distal venous arterialization as a lower limb salvage proce-dure. Am Surg 2011;77(6):726–30.
19. Schreve MA, Minnee RC, Bosma J, et al. Compara-tive study of venous arterialization and pedal bypass in a patient cohort with critical limb ischemia. Ann Vasc Surg 2014;28(5):1123–7.
20. King TA, Marks J, Berrettoni BA, et al. Arteriovenous reversal for limb salvage in unreconstructible upper extremity arterial occlusive disease. J Vasc Surg 1993;17(5):924–32.
21. Kind GM. Arterialization of the venous system of the hand. Plast Reconstr Surg 2006;118(2):421–8.
22. Matarrese MR, Hammert WC. Revascularization of the ischemic hand with arterialization of the venous system. J Hand Surg Am 2011;36(12):2047–51.
23. Pokrovsky AV, Dan VN, Chupin AV, et al. Arterializa-tion of the hand venous system in patients with critical ischemia and thrombangiitis obliterans. Angiol Sosud Khir 2007;13(2):105–11 [in English, Russian].
24. Chloros GD, Li Z, Koman LA. Long-term successful outcome of severe hand ischemia using arterializa-tion with reversal of venous flow: case report. J Hand Surg Am 2008;33(7):1048–51.
25. Pederson WC. Revascularization of the chronically ischemic hand. Hand Clin 1999;15(4):629–42.
26. Oishi SN, Levin LS, Pederson WC. Microsurgical management of extremity wounds in diabetics with peripheral vascular disease. Plast Reconstr Surg 1993;92(3):485–92.
27. Malikov S, Magnan PE, Casanova D, et al. Bypass flap reconstruction, a novel technique for distal revascularization: outcome of first 10 clinical cases. Ann Vasc Surg 2009;23(6):745–52.
28. Serletti JM, Hurwitz SR, Jones JA, et al. Extension of limb salvage by combined vascular reconstruction and adjunctive free-tissue transfer. J Vasc Surg 1993;18(6):972–8.
29. Horch RE, Lang W, Arkudas A, et al. Nutrient free flaps with vascular bypasses for extremity salvage in patients with chronic limb ischemia. J Cardiovasc Surg (Torino) 2014;55(2 Suppl 1):265–72.
30. Goldsmith HS, Griffith AL, Kupferman A, et al. Lipid angiogenic factor from omentum. JAMA 1984; 252(15):2034–6.

31. Garcia-Gomez I, Goldsmith HS, Angulo J, et al. Angiogenic capacity of human omental stem cells. Neurol Res 2005;27(8):807–11.

32. Bhat MA, Zaroo MI, Darzi MA. Omental transplantation for critical limb ischemia in Buerger's disease. Plast Reconstr Surg 2007;119(6):1979–80.

33. Nishimura A, Sano F, Nakanishi Y, et al. Omental transplantation for relief of limb ischemia. Surg Forum 1977;28:213–5.

34. Singh I, Ramteke VK. The role of omental transfer in Buerger's disease: New Delhi's experience. Aust N Z J Surg 1996;66(6):372–6.

35. Herrera HR, Geary J, Whitehead P, et al. Revascularization of the lower extremity with omentum. Clin Plast Surg 1991;18(3):491–5.

36. Ala-Kulju K, Virkkula L. Use of omental pedicle for treatment of Buerger's disease affecting the upper extremities. A modified technique. Vasa 1990;19(4):330–3.

37. Zaha H, Inamine S. Laparoscopically harvested omental flap: results for 96 patients. Surg Endosc 2010;24(1):103–7.

38. Horch RE, Horbach T, Lang W. The nutrient omentum free flap: revascularization with vein bypasses and greater omentum flap in severe arterial ulcers. J Vasc Surg 2007;45(4):837–40.

39. Goldsmith HS. The omentum: research and clinical applications. 1st edition. New York: Springer Verlag; 1990.

40. Maloney CT Jr, Wages D, Upton J, et al. Free omental tissue transfer for extremity coverage and revascularization. Plast Reconstr Surg 2003;111(6): 1899–904.

41. Sultanov DD, Gaibov AD, Kurbatov UA, et al. Revascularization in distal lesions of upper extremity arteries. Angiol Sosud Khir 2005;11(4):117–23 [in English, Russian].

Options for Revascularization: Artery Versus Vein: Technical Considerations

John Shuck, MD[a], Derek L. Masden, MD[a,b],*

KEYWORDS

- Upper extremity bypass • Upper extremity revascularization • Arterial conduits • Arterial grafts

KEY POINTS

- Vascular grafts, as either interpositional conduits or bypass grafts, can be used for revascularization procedures in the upper extremity.
- Vein grafts are more readily available and can be easier to harvest.
- Arterial grafts may provide superior patency rates compared with vein grafts.
- Arterial grafts can be located and harvested with consistent and reliable anatomy throughout the body.

INTRODUCTION

Vascular reconstructions, in the form of interposition conduits or bypass grafts, are often needed for definitive management of upper-extremity ischemia. Indications for reconstruction include both isolated lesions resulting from repetitive trauma or use (eg, hypothenar hammer syndrome) and a multitude of systemic disease with upper-extremity vascular manifestations. Such systemic diseases include collagen vascular disease (scleroderma, CREST [calcinosis, Raynaud's phenomenon, esophageal dysmotility, sclerodactyly and telangiectasia], lupus erythematosis), Buerger disease, advanced renal disease, diabetes, and peripheral vascular disease.[1] Following adequate excision of the diseased segments, primary end-to-end closure is often not possible, necessitating interpositional grafts. Alternatively, the diseased segment may be left in situ with end-to-side bypass grafting, providing an alternate avenue for perfusion to the end tissues.

ARTERIAL VERSUS VENOUS GRAFTS
Flow Dynamics and Intimal Hyperplasia

Historically, vein grafts have been the mainstay of treatment given their widespread availability and ease of harvest. Vein grafts are most commonly accomplished with reversed vein grafts harvested from the ipsilateral arm (superficial venous system) or the leg (greater or lesser saphenous veins). More recently, arterial grafts have gained popularity given the concern for high rates of vein graft occlusion postoperatively. Alterations in flow dynamics following vein grafting may result in intermediate and long-term graft occlusion. Several studies have demonstrated adaptive intimal hyperplasia that results when vein grafts are subjected to arterial flow and subsequent intimal sheer stress. The end result is luminal narrowing in up to 30% to 50% of patients.[2,3] In accordance with the reconstructive principle of "replacing like with like," arterial grafts provide native vessels more aptly suited to the high-pressure system

The authors have nothing to disclose.

a Department of Plastic Surgery, Georgetown University Hospital, 3800 Reservoir Road, Washington, DC 20007, USA; b Division of Plastic Surgery, Hand Surgery, Washington Hospital Center, 106 Irving Street Northwest, POB 420 South, Washington, DC 20010, USA
* Corresponding author. Division of Plastic Surgery, Hand Surgery, Washington Hospital Center, 106 Irving Street Northwest, POB 420 South, Washington, DC 20010.
E-mail address: derekmasden@gmail.com

0749-0712/15/$ – see front matter © 2015 Elsevier Inc. All rights reserved.

with reduced compensatory intimal hyperplasia.[4] The use of arterial grafts for peripheral bypass has been studied extensively in the vascular surgery literature since the 1960s.[5] Much of the recent focus on arterial bypass grafts is based on cardiac surgery literature in which patency and success rates have been shown to be superior in the setting of coronary artery bypass grafting.[4]

In Situ Graft Vasodilatory Response and Growth

There is some evidence that arterial grafts continue to respond to local vasodilatory (strong response) and vasocontrictive (weak response) mediators; this has been demonstrated with the deep inferior epigastric artery (DIEA) in vitro.[6] Furthermore, work by Faruqui and Stoney[5] indicates that arterial grafts in children continue to grow proportionally following inset. The authors find this property to be unique to arterial grafts.[5] Although these studies may be considered investigational, such data do support the hypothesis that arteries are truly the more physiologic graft compared with their venous counterparts. Finally, a recent systematic review of the literature noted arterial grafts have higher patency rates postoperatively than do venous grafts when used for upper-extremity vascular reconstruction.[7]

Anatomical Variations in Arterial Versus Venous Grafts

From an anatomic standpoint, arterial grafts are better suited to upper-extremity bypass when compared with veins. Within the hand, narrow outflow vessels with numerous branch points require multiple distal outflow junctures; this has become increasingly relevant as revascularization techniques have evolved and a more extensive surgical exploration of the hand has become standard. Although earlier reconstructions relied on single-vessel exposures and isolated segment excision (radial or ulnar arteries), now more aggressive identification of the superficial arch as well as both common and proper digital vessels have become commonplace.[8,9] This approach allows for a more thorough assessment of disease and identification of healthy outflow arterial targets. As such, there is often a need for a conduit or graft that allows revascularization of multiple, small-caliber outflow vessels. Venous grafts must be reversed in situ (unless a valvulotome is used) to prevent the native valve from impeding flow. A significant size mismatch is often encountered when vein grafts are reversed; this is of particular concern with anastomoses distal to the wrist.

In addition, reversed vein grafts rarely provide usable branches for revascularizing multiple small distal outflow arteries. In contrast, arterial grafts maintain the proximal to distal orientation, allowing for excellent size matching distally. Several commonly used arterial grafts also end in multiple small distal branches, ideally suited for anastomosis to the digital arteries (**Fig. 1**). These side branches can also be used in small vessel revascularization, such as digital replant or revascularization requiring interpositional grafts.

Last, the handling and microsurgical anastomosis of an artery to artery can be less challenging and less prone to technical errors than veins because of their thicker wall with less tendency to collapse.

Indications for Venous Grafts

Despite the potential superiority of arterial grafts in upper-extremity vascular reconstruction, there are certain scenarios in which the surgeon must consider using a vein. The most common of such indications is the need for significant length. The most commonly used arterial grafts offer only 10 to 15 cm in length at most. However, when the reconstructive surgeon is confronted with gaps or diseased segments in excess of 20 cm, often a long venous graft must be used.

In addition, venous grafts are often superficial, lending to an easier exposure and harvest compared with their arterial counterparts, which often require deeper and more tedious dissections. It is also possible to harvest a vein graft from the ipsilateral arm, reducing the surgical burden to the patient. Any of the arterial graft options require surgical exploration of an additional extremity or the trunk, resulting in an additional donor site and morbidity.

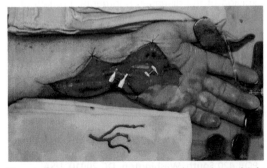

Fig. 1. Thoracodorsal arterial graft with multiple distal branches prepared for inset. (*From* Masden DL, McClinton MA. Arterial conduits for distal upper extremity bypass. J Hand Surg Am 2013;38(3):572–7; with permission.)

Preoperative Evaluation

Preoperatively, a thorough history and physical examination should be performed to identify previous operations and/or scars that may have damaged or transected potential arterial donors. Preoperative imaging may also aid in identifying the availability of donors. Imaging may include CT angiography/MR angiography for abdominal or thigh vessels (DIEA or descending femoral circumflex artery system). Duplex ultrasound is also a helpful adjunct for determining patency and caliber of the greater and lesser saphenous veins.

Last, the commonly used arterial grafts also serve as main pedicles for both workhorse fasciocutaneous and musculocutaneous reconstructive flaps. Therefore, harvest of these vessels precludes the use of their native flap territories for future soft tissue reconstruction; this is of particular concern in the case of significant soft tissue trauma requiring both revascularization and soft tissue flap coverage.

ARTERIAL GRAFTS
Background

Given adequate collateral flow, any artery may be used as an arterial graft for upper-extremity revascularization. The trunk is privileged with a rich network of interconnecting angiosomes. Even in patients with peripheral vascular disease, advanced renal disease, or diabetes, sufficient collateral flow enables harvest of uninvolved arteries in the trunk. However, for the upper-extremity surgeon, this may be foreign territory anatomically. Generally speaking, the arterial pedicles of commonly used flaps for free tissue transfers make for excellent grafts and conduits. Selection of common free flap pedicles minimizes donor site morbidity and may be easily compensated for by surrounding collateral flow. Numerous donor arteries have been described

and in theory any artery that can be sacrificed without significant consequence or is redundant can be viewed as a potential graft. Most commonly used are the DIEA, lateral circumflex femoral artery, or the thoracodorsal artery for elective arterial grafting.

Deep Inferior Epigastric Artery
Anatomy

Originating at the external iliac artery, the DIEA travels superomedially in the preperitoneal plane and anastomoses with the superior epigastric artery in the rectus abdominis muscle. The DIEA enters the underside of the rectus abdominis muscle laterally 10 cm above the pubic symphysis. The DIEA reliably provides 12 cm of length over 1 mm in diameter. The diameter at its origin is generally 2.5 to 3.5 mm. As the vessel enters the rectus muscle, diameters of 1 to 2 mm are encountered.[10–13]

Surgical harvest

Exposure may be achieved via a longitudinal paramedian incision directly over the vessel's native course as described above. In the thin and moderately sized patient, the rectus may be palpated. An infraumbilical incision is performed over the lateral rectus border, gently curving laterally at a point approximately 10 cm above the pubic symphysis. The lateral curve should bisect the pubis and the anterior superior iliac spine and may be directed toward the palpable femoral pulse (**Fig. 2**A). Dissection is carried down through the subcutaneous fat until the fascia is encountered. A small fascial incision can be made to confirm correct location at the lateral recuts border. Rectus muscle fibers run vertically. One should be cautious of the obese or multiparous female patient, as significant diastasis causes wide splaying and lateral migration of the rectus muscles. The fascia may be incised along its length with care taken to preserve an adequate

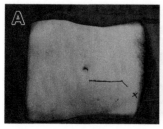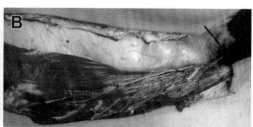

Fig. 2. (*A*) Markings for the skin incision for the DIEA harvest. (*B*) Cadaver dissection showing DIEA branching from the external iliac artery (*arrow*) to lie on the posterior aspect of the rectus abdominis muscle. (*From* Masden DL, McClinton MA. Arterial conduits for distal upper extremity bypass. J Hand Surg Am 2013;38(3):572–7; with permission.)

cuff both medially and laterally for closure. The rectus muscle is then gently swept medially to reveal the vessels lateral to the muscle (see **Fig. 2**B). Inferiorly, the vessel is encased in loose areolar fat, which may be easily dissected. Vasodilatory agents such as papaverine are useful in preventing vasospasm during harvest. Numerous small side branches are encountered. These branches may be dissected and left long before ligation if multiple digital vessel reconstruction is planned.

Donor site morbidity

The main donor site complications of DIEA harvest may be attributed to weakening of the abdominal wall. Therefore, there is a risk of both hernia and lower abdominal bulge. Proper technique should minimize both. Care should be taken to provide meticulous anterior sheath closure.

Descending Branch of the Lateral Circumflex Femoral Artery

Anatomy

Following bifurcation from the common femoral artery, the profunda femoris gives off the lateral circumflex femoral artery. This large-caliber vessel runs deep to the sartorius and rectus femoris in the proximal thigh, giving off 3 main vessels: the ascending, descending, and transverse branches. The descending branch is consistently found running inferiorly in the interval between the vastus lateralis laterally and the rectus femoris medially. The floor of this intermuscular septum is the vasuts intermedius. The artery travels most commonly with 2 venae commitantes as well as the motor nerves to the vastus lateralis and rectus femoris. The descending branch of the lateral circumflex femoral artery is the main pedicle for the anterolateral thigh (ALT) flap. Its reliability and consistency has made the ALT a workhorse flap for many reconstructive surgeons. Harvestable length is 10 to 15 cm with average vessel diameter of 2 to 3 mm.[14,15]

Surgical harvest

In thin patients, the intermuscular septum between the vastus lateralis and rectus femoris may be visualized on the skin surface. In patients in whom the septum is not readily apparent on the lateral thigh, estimation and incision planning are easily accomplished using the following landmarks. A straight line is drawn connecting the anterior superior iliac spine to the lateral border of the patella (**Fig. 3**A). The incision for harvest is then made along the middle third of this line. The fascia is incised, revealing the intermuscular septum between the vastus lateralis and the recuts femoris. The surgeon may confirm the correct interval by examining the underside of the suspected rectus femoris medially. The underbelly of the rectus femoris muscle in this region is distinct "salmon-skin" silver. Gentle separation of the muscles with the aid of a deep self-retaining retractor will reveal the vessel (see **Fig. 3**B).

Dissection of the descending branch can then proceed in a distal to proximal fashion. The motor nerves will be identified traveling in parallel and should be carefully preserved. The artery will give off several perforating branches in both a septocutaneous and a musculocutaneous fashion. These branches can be dissected and used for digital artery anastomosis in the hand.[16] Occasionally, the descending branch enters the vastus lateralis distally and may require intramuscular dissection. The proximal dissection may be carried up to its origin from the lateral circumflex femoral artery.

Donor site morbidity

Injury to the native motor and sensory nerves in the lateral thigh is the biggest drawback to harvest of the descending branch of the lateral femoral circumflex artery. However, careful surgical technique and knowledge of the local anatomy minimize this risk. Injury to the lateral femoral cutaneous nerve can cause neuralgias of the lateral thigh. In addition, injury to the motor nerves to the vastus lateralis or rectus femoris may cause

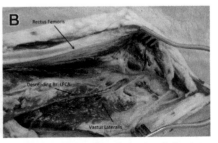
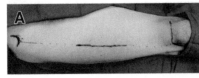

Fig. 3. (*A*) Markings for the skin incision for the harvest of the descending branch of the lateral circumflex femoral artery along the intermuscular septum. (*B*) Cadaver dissection showing descending branch of the lateral circumflex femoral artery between the vastus lateralis and rectus femoris. (*From* Masden DL, McClinton MA. Arterial conduits for distal upper extremity bypass. J Hand Surg Am 2013;38(3):572–7; with permission.)

muscle weakness. Hematoma and seroma may be minimized by performing layered closure over closed-suction drains.

Thoracodorsal or Subscapular System

Anatomy

Another workhorse reconstructive flap well-suited for arterial conduit harvest is the latissimus dorsi muscle. The arterial pedicle has extremely consistent anatomy that affords both excellent caliber and length. Deep within the axilla, the axillary artery gives off the subscapular artery from its third segment.[17] Approximately 2 cm from its origin, the subscapular artery gives off the circumflex scapular artery that travels posteriorly over the scapula bone. The subscapular artery then continues inferiorly and becomes the thoracodorsal artery. The thoracodorsal runs approximately 1 to 2 cm medial and parallel to the lateral border of the latissimus muscle in a vertical direction. With the exception of the morbidly obese patient, the lateral border of the latissimus muscle can be easily palpated in most patients. A pencil Doppler will reveal a strong signal coursing 1 to 2 cm medial to this border. The thoracodorsal artery gives off 1 or 2 proximal branches to the serratus. The thoracodorsal proper then bifurcates into 2 intramuscular branches. The descending branch continues along the lateral border of the latissimus, while the transverse branch proceeds medially paralleling the superior border of the muscle. An arterial graft approximately 11 cm in length with a proximal diameter as large as 1 to 2 cm may be harvested.

Surgical harvest

Harvest of the thoracodorsal artery can be undertaken in either the supine or the lateral decubitus position. Preparing the arm into the field allows for active abduction and movement of the arm, thereby facilitating dissection. Anterior to the posterior axillary fold, a vertical zigzag or transverse incision is made (**Fig. 4**A). The lateral/anterior border of the latissimus muscle is identified. The dissection is then carried deep anterior to the muscle border. Initial identification of the thoracodorsal is sometimes obscured by local fatty tissue. The use of the pencil Doppler facilitates identification. Once identified, the vessel can be easily traced both proximally into the axilla and distally along its course parallel the latissimus edge. Proximally, the dissection can be carried up to the branch point of the circumflex scapular artery, approximately 2 to 3 cm from the subscapular artery's origin from the axillary artery. The use of lighted retraction and careful dissection minimizes the risk of large-vessel injury and damage to the thoracodorsal nerve. Distally, the branches to the serratus anterior may be identified and harvested if needed. If dissection and harvest of the serratus branch are performed, one must take care not to injure the long thoracic nerve running along the chest wall to the serratus (see **Fig. 4**B). On the underside of the latissimus, the descending and transverse branches of the thoracodorsal artery may be dissected intramuscularly if needed. The secondary blood supply to the latissimus comes from thoracolumbar perforators in the lower back. These vessels prevent muscle ischemia following harvest of its dominant arterial pedicle.

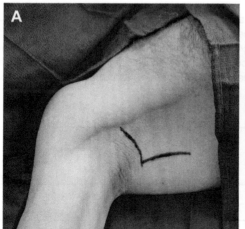
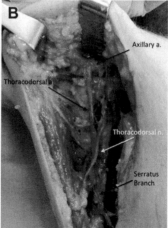

Fig. 4. (*A*) Markings for the harvest of the thoracodorsal artery. (*B*) Cadaver dissection showing thoracodorsal artery as the terminal aspect of the subscapular arterial system. (*From* Masden DL, McClinton MA. Arterial conduits for distal upper extremity bypass. J Hand Surg Am 2013;38(3):572–7; with permission.)

Donor site morbidity

Injury to the motor nerve of the latissimus can result in functional deficit at the shoulder. In addition, seroma formation following dissection in this area is notoriously problematic. Again, using meticulous layered closure and judicious placement of closed-suction drains may minimize this complication.

Superficial Inferior Epigastric Artery

The superficial inferior epigastric artery (SIEA) would be an ideal donor graft if not for its notoriously unpredictable and often absent course. Its superficial location in the lower abdomen makes for easy dissection compared with most arterial grafts. However, the average usable length is only around 6 cm with an average diameter of 1.4 mm, although it is exquisitely sensitive to manipulation and vasospasm (**Table 1**). The SIEA has been shown to be absent in 35% of the population.[18–20] As such, it is not a reliable option and its use should be considered only if it is encountered during the exposure for the DIEA.

VENOUS GRAFTS

More expendable than arteries, venous grafts can be harvested from virtually anywhere in the body without consequence. The most common venous grafts used for upper extremity include the cephalic and basilic veins in the arm and the greater and lesser saphenous veins in the leg. Their superficial subcutaneous location facilitates easy exposure without much risk for morbidity. Exposure and harvest techniques for these veins are well described because of their frequent use in peripheral vascular disease and coronary artery disease surgery.

If these veins are not available or are inadequate, it is possible to use veins from the deeper systems. All of the potential arterial grafts described previously travel with 1 to 3 venae comitants that are of similar caliber. These deeper veins are often spared from disease and can provide venous grafts. One of the authors' preferred donors is the vena comitans of the posterior tibial artery. These veins are found in the medial aspect of the lower leg, in the plane between the soleus and the deep posterior compartment. If exposure of the greater saphenous vein proves to be inadequate, it is easy to convert to a deeper dissection through the fascia, exposing the posterior tibial system.

HAND/RECIPIENT VESSEL PREPARATION
Graft/Conduit Inset

Preparation of the recipient vessels in the hand is performed similarly for either a venous or an arterial conduit. As discussed previously, the authors tend to favor more extensive exposure to ensure adequate identification and excision of diseased segments to effectively perform anastomoses "outside of the zone of injury." A strongly positive "spurt test" as well as vessel resection proximal to a patent side branch assures adequate inflow. The lumen and intima of the inflow/outflow targets are carefully assessed for trauma and clot formation under the operating microscope. Once the gap is carefully measured, the arterial or venous conduit is then planned. The main difference between arterial and venous grafts is the planned length. Following anastomosis and return of flow, venous grafts tend to lengthen, whereas arterial grafts maintain their inset length. For this reason, arterial grafts are generally constructed using the exact gap length, whereas venous grafts are slightly shorter and sutured in under mild stretch, preventing redundancy and potential kinking following return of inflow.

Vasospasm

Vasospasm not only can result in local tissue ischemia but also may alter laminar flow and propagate thrombus. Therefore, every effort must be undertaken to reduce local vasospasm during

Table 1 Arterial donor graft dimensions		
Arterial Graft	**Length, Avg. (Range)**	**Diameter, Avg. (Range)**
DIEA	16 (14–18)	3.5 (3–4)
SIEA	6 (4–8)	4 (3–5)
Descending branch of the lateral circumflex artery	12 (8–16)	2.1 (2–5)
Thoracodorsal artery	8.5 (6.5–12)	3 (2–4)
Subscapular artery	20 (10–24)	1.2 (0.8–1.2)

Table 2
Artery/vein graft patency rate by study

Study Authors, Year	Artery/Vein	Patients	Grafts	Follow-up (mo)	Patency (%)
Temming et al,[15] 2011	A	2	3	18	100
Lifchez et al, 2009[21]	V	12	12	52	66.7
Chloros et al, 2008[22]	V	12	13	54	76.9
Rockwell et al,[20] 2007	A	8	9	12	100
Namdari et al, 2007[23]	V	3	3	9	100
Duene et al, 2005[24]	V	1	1	12	100
Dethmers et al,[17] 2005	V	3	3	43	100
Dethmers et al,[17] 2005	A/V	23	24	43	79.2
Smith et al, 2004[25]	A	3	3	16	100
Rockwell et al,[19] 2003	A	1	1	12	100
Ruch et al, 2000[26]	V	13	13	22	100
Ferris et al, 2000[27]	V	19	19	22	84.2
Zimmerman et al, 1994[28]	V	8	8	40	87.5
Nehler et al, 1992[29]	V	15	17	14	94.1
Barral et al, 1992[30]	V	8	8	66	75
Mehlhoff et al, 1991[31]	V	8	8	66	87.5
Harris et al, 1990[32]	V	6	7	24	100

graft harvest and inset. The first and perhaps most important factor affecting vessel spasm is the application of meticulous microsurgical technique. This meticulous microsurgical technique includes careful vessel handling and avoidance of intimal damage at all costs. Intraluminal placement of micro-forceps should be minimized with adventitial grasping used sparingly only when necessary. Application of both local and systemic vasodilatory agents is useful. Papaverine is applied to the grafts periodically and following clamp removal. In the absence of allergies and/or medical contraindications, calcium channel blockers are administered postoperatively.

Patency Outcomes

Early reporting on outcomes using arterial grafts for upper-extremity bypass are favorable when compared with their venous counterparts. Intermediate term outcomes show patency rates of up to 100% at follow-up (**Table 2**).[7]

To date, no long-term outcome studies have been published in the setting of upper-extremity bypass. However, the relative ease of handling and inset afforded by arterial conduits may outweigh the added time required for surgical harvest. The use of arterial donors for vascular grafts and conduits in the upper extremity is the authors' preference. A thorough knowledge of available arterial donors allows the upper-extremity surgeon an alternative option for vascular reconstruction.

REFERENCES

1. Jones NF. Acute and chronic ischemia of the hand: pathophysiology, treatment, and prognosis. J Hand Surg Am 1991;16(6):1074–83.
2. Owens CD. Adaptive changes in autogenous vein grafts for arterial reconstruction: clinical implications. J Vasc Surg 2010;51(3):736–46.
3. McCann RL, Hagen PO, Fuchs JC. Aspirin and dipyridamole decrease intimal hyperplasia in experimental vein grafts. Ann Surg 1980;191(2):238–43.
4. Cooper GJ, Underwood MJ, Deverall PB. Arterial and venous conduits for coronary artery bypass. A current review. Eur J Cardiothorac Surg 1996; 10(2):129–40.
5. Faruqui RM, Stoney RJ. The arterial autograft. In: Cronenwett JL, Gloviczki P, Johnston KW, et al, editors. Rutherford vascular surgery. 5th edition. Philadelphia: WB Saunders; 2000. p. 532–9.
6. Mugge A, Barton MR, Cremer J, et al. Different vascular reactivity of human internal mammary and inferior epigastric arteries in vitro. Ann Thorac Surg 1993;56(5):1085–9.
7. Masden DL, Seruya M, Higgins P. A systematic review of the outcomes of distal upper extremity bypass surgery with arterial and venous conduits. J Hand Surg Am 2012;37(11):2362–7.

8. Masden DL, McClinton MA. Arterial conduits for distal upper extremity bypass. J Hand Surg Am 2013;38(3):572–7.

9. Koman LA, Ruch DS, Peterson-Smith B, et al. Vascular disorders. In: Green DP, Hotchkiss RN, Pederson WC, et al, editors. Green's operative hand surgery. 5th edition. Philadelphia: Elsevier Churchill Livingstone; 2005. p. 2265–313.

10. Taylor GI, Daniel RK. The anatomy of several free flap donor sites. Plast Reconstr Surg 1975;56(3): 243–53.

11. Zenn MR, Pribaz J, Walsh M. Use of the descending lateral femoral circumflex artery and vein for vascular grafting: a better alternative to an arteriovenous loop. Plast Reconstr Surg 2010;126(1):140–2.

12. Fabbrocini M, Fattouch K, Camporini G, et al. The descending branch of lateral femoral circumflex artery in arterial CABG: early and midterm results. Ann Thorac Surg 2003;75(6):1836–41.

13. Park JH, Min KH, Eun SC, et al. Scalp free flap reconstruction using anterolateral thigh flap pedicle for interposition artery and vein grafts. Arch Plast Surg 2012;39(1):55–8.

14. Bianchi B, Copelli C, Ferrari S, et al. Anterolateral thigh flap pedicle for interposition artery and vein grafts in head and neck reconstruction: a case report. Microsurgery 2009;29(2):136–7.

15. Temming JF, van Uchelen JH, Tellier MA. Hypothenar hammer syndrome: distal ulnar artery reconstruction with autologous descending branch of the lateral circumflex femoral artery. Tech Hand Up Extrem Surg 2011;15(1):24–7.

16. Mathes SJ, Nahai F. Latissimus dorsi flap. In: Mathes SJ, Nahai F, editors. Reconstructive surgery: principles, anatomy, & technique. New York: Churchhill Livingstone; 1997. p. 565–615.

17. Dethmers RS, Houpt P. Surgical management of hypothenar and thenar hammer syndromes: a retrospective study of 31 instances in 28 patients. J Hand Surg 2005;30B(4):419–23.

18. Mathes SJ, Nahai F. Superficial inferior epigastric artery (SIEA) flap. In: Mathes SJ, Nahai F, editors. Reconstructive surgery: principles, anatomy, & technique. New York: Churchill Livingstone; 1997. p. 1095–105.

19. Rockwell WB, Smith SM, Tolliston T, et al. Arterial conduits for extremity microvascular bypass surgery. Plast Reconstr Surg 2003;112(3):829–34.

20. Rockwell WB, Hurst CA, Morton DA, et al. The deep inferior epigastric artery: anatomy and applicability as a source of microvascular arterial grafts. Plast Reconstr Surg 2007;120(1):209–14.

21. Lifchez SD, Higgins JP. Long-term results of surgical treatment for hypothenar hammer syndrome. Plast Reconstr Surg 2009;124:210–6.

22. Chloros GD, Li Z, Koman LA. Long-term successful outcome of severe hand ischemia using arterialization with reversal of venous flow: case report. J Hand Surg 2008;33A:1048–51.

23. Namdari S, Weiss AP, Carney WI Jr. Palmar bypass for digital ischemia. J Hand Surg 2007;32A:1251–8.

24. Deune EG, McCarthy EF. Reconstruction of a true ulnar artery aneurysm in a 4-year-old patient with radial artery agenesis. Orthopedics 2005;28:1459–61.

25. Smith HE, Dirks M, Patterson RB. Hypothenar hammer syndrome: Distal ulnar artery reconstruction with autologous inferior epigastric artery. J Vasc Surg 2004;40:1238–42.

26. Ruch DS, Aldridge M, Holden M, et al. Arterial reconstruction for radial artery occlusion. J Hand Surg 2000;25A:282–90.

27. Ferris BL, Taylor LM Jr, Oyama K, et al. Hypothenar hammer syndrome: proposed etiology. J Vasc Surg 2000;31:104–13.

28. Zimmerman NB, Zimmerman SI, McClinton MA, et al. Long-term recovery following surgical treatment for ulnar artery occlusion. J Hand Surg 1994; 19A:17–21.

29. Nehler MR, Dalman RL, Harris EJ, et al. Upper extremity arterial bypass distal to the wrist. J Vasc Surg 1992;16:633–40.

30. Barral X, Favre JP, Gournier JP, et al. Late results of palmar arch bypass in the treatment of digital trophic disorders. Ann Vasc Surg 1992;6:418–24.

31. Mehlhoff TL, Wood MB. Ulnar artery thrombosis and the role of interposition vein grafting: patency with microsurgical technique. J Hand Surg 1991;16A:274–8.

32. Harris EJ Jr, Taylor LM Jr, Edwards JM, et al. Surgical treatment of distal ulnar artery aneurysm. Am J Surg 1990;159:527–30.

Complications Related to Radial Artery Occlusion, Radial Artery Harvest, and Arterial Lines

Harvey Chim, MD[a], Karim Bakri, MBBS[b],
Steven L. Moran, MD[b],*

KEYWORDS

- Radial artery occlusion • Hand ischemia • Transradial catheterization • Radial forearm flap
- Radial artery

KEY POINTS

- Hemodynamic changes occur within the forearm and hand following sacrifice of the radial artery.
- Complications in cases of transradial catheterization can be minimized with proper patient selection, the use of heparin, and the technique of patent hemostasis.
- Radial artery occlusion and distal ischemia in cases of indwelling radial catheters can result in tissue loss and amputation.

INTRODUCTION

Owing to its superficial location, the radial artery has been a popular choice for the placement of arterial lines, and is increasingly becoming the standard access option for cannulation in cases of cardiac catheterization.[1] In a similar fashion, the radial artery forearm flap has been a workhorse as a free flap and pedicled flap for reconstruction of the upper extremity because of its reliable blood supply and ease of harvest. The presumed expendability of the radial artery was based on early anatomic studies by Coleman and Anson[2] that demonstrated the larger size of the ulnar artery at the level of the wrist and its dominant supply to the superficial palmar arch, and, by assumption, the entire hand. Recent studies have questioned these findings, and have found that in certain circumstances the radial artery is actually the larger artery at the level of the wrist. Riekkinen and colleagues[3] found, in a cadaveric study of arterial

diameter, that the mean diameter of the radial artery was 28% larger than the ulnar artery in the right arm and 26% larger than the ulnar artery in the left arm. Other studies have found that the size of the radial artery may depend on many factors including gender, smoking status, and the presence of hypertension or hyperlipidemia.[4,5]

Proper selection of patients for radial artery harvest, radial catheterization, or radial forearm flap harvest is critical. Patient screening for such procedures has traditionally been performed through an Allen test. The Allen test is performed by occluding the radial and ulnar artery at the level of the wrist and then evaluating hand perfusion through observed restoration of capillary refill after selective release of the ulnar artery. The time frame for safe return of perfusion is an arbitrary threshold that has been set at between 5 and 9 seconds.[6] A normal Allen test implies the presence of a complete ulnopalmar arch. A patent and complete

The authors have nothing to disclose.
[a] Division of Plastic Surgery, University of Miami Medical Center, 1600 Northwest 10th Avenue #1140, Miami, FL 33136, USA; [b] Division of Plastic Surgery, Mayo Clinic, 200 First Street Southwest, Rochester, MN 55905, USA
* Corresponding author.
E-mail address: Moran.steven@mayo.edu

0749-0712/15/$ – see front matter © 2015 Elsevier Inc. All rights reserved.

hand.theclinics.com

arch should allow for perfusion of the thumb and fingers following harvest or occlusion of the radial artery; however, an Allen test does not take into account the presence of noncritical stenosis or occlusive lesions in the digital arteries or in the ulnar artery itself, which may manifest clinically over time following harvest of the radial artery.[7] Whereas some studies have reported that the Allen test is reliable in selecting patients for radial artery harvest, others have questioned its reliability and have advocated for more objective tests such as photoplethysmography, direct digit pressure measurement, or Doppler ultrasonography in conjunction with the Allen test.[6,8–11] Adequate blood flow despite an abnormal Allen test could include augmented inflow through the anterior interosseous artery or through a persistent median artery, which has a reported incidence of 20%.[12]

Greenwood and colleagues[13] found that patients with abnormal Allen tests tended to be male, with larger-diameter radial arteries at the level of the wrist in comparison with those who had a normal Allen test. In addition, patients with abnormal Allen test were found to have elevated thumb lactate levels after only 30 minutes of radial artery occlusion (RAO). Greenwood's conclusion was that any patient with an abnormal Allen test should not undergo transradial cardiac catheterization because of the risks of subsequent hand ischemia if RAO were to occur.

In the classic 1985 article by Jones and O'Brien,[14] acute hand ischemia was reported following elevation of a radial forearm flap in a patient with a normal Allen test. This case report started the debate as to whether all radial arteries should be reconstructed following radial forearm flap harvest. Similar case reports have been reported since, strengthening such concerns; however, more concerning is Varley and colleagues'[15] report of acute hand ischemia 4 weeks following elevation of a radial forearm flap in a patient with a normal Allen test and a normal Doppler ultrasonogram preoperatively. When raising a radial forearm flap, the authors' method is to occlude the radial artery at the level of the wrist before dividing the radial artery with a vascular clamp. The tourniquet is then released and thumb perfusion is verified before dividing the artery and completing flap elevation. Although case reports of acute hand ischemia are rare, it still heightens one's awareness for the potential dangers associated with radial artery harvest and has led investigators to examine which compensatory changes occur within the hand and forearm following removal or occlusion of the radial artery.

COMPENSATORY CHANGES FOLLOWING RADIAL ARTERY HARVEST

With sacrifice of the radial artery, the flow in other arteries in the forearms increases to compensate. A statistically significant increase in blood flow has been documented within the ulnar, posterior interosseous, and anterior interosseous arteries using color duplex imaging following harvest of a radial forearm flap.[16] An increase in ulnar artery diameter and flow rate has also been reported 3 months after harvest of the radial artery, with increased flow seen in the ulnar artery after ischemic forearm exercise.[17] These compensatory changes have been found to result in normal hand perfusion in the immediate postoperative period, with normal digital-brachial indices, cold response, grip and pinch strength, and 2-point discrimination.[18] Meland and colleagues[19] found, in a study of 13 consecutive free radial forearm flaps, that at an average of 6 months' follow-up patients had no demonstrable differences in transcutaneous oxygen levels, digital-brachial blood pressure indices, and cutaneous blood flow as measured by laser flow Doppler when compared with the contralateral "normal" side. Such findings do not support the routine reconstruction of the radial artery following elevation of the radial forearm flap.

Despite these short-term results, longer periods of follow-up have pointed to changes within the hemodynamics of the forearm and hand after harvest of the radial artery. Exercise intolerance with decrease in tissue oxygenation of the affected hand has been reported 1 year after radial artery harvest.[20] Serial Doppler evaluation of the ulnar artery has found increases in peak systolic velocity and thickness of the intima of the ulnar artery following radial artery harvest. In addition, there is an increased prevalence of atherosclerotic plaques in both the ulnar artery and asymptomatic hand ischemia 10 years after radial artery harvest.[21–23] Using pulse volume recording plethysmography, Lee and colleagues[24] reported an overall decrease in blood flow to all fingers of the operated arm after harvest of the radial artery. The same investigators reported that the digital blood flow eventually improves as a result of increased flow through the ulnar artery.[25] Other studies have reported no increased incidence of atherosclerotic plaques in the ulnar artery at late follow-up, but with increased peak systolic velocity in the ulnar artery long-term sequelae are still unknown.[26,27] Hence the late hand and forearm morbidity following radial artery harvest may also depend on the overall health and comorbidities of the individual patient.

A single case of acute hypothenar hammer syndrome has been reported in a laborer several years following a radial forearm flap harvest.[28] This patient presented 4.5 years after harvest of a radial forearm flap for elbow coverage, with cold intolerance and necrosis in the pulp of the long and ring fingers. The patient worked in a high-risk occupation as a plumber and used his hand as a hammer to test plumbing. The patient required ulnar artery reconstruction with an interposition saphenous vein graft for salvage of the fingers and thumb. In considering whether the radial artery should be sacrificed, the occupation of the patient and the possibility of high-risk behavior should be carefully considered.

COMPLICATIONS FOLLOWING TRANSRADIAL CATHETERIZATION AND CANNULATION
Transradial Catheterization

The radial artery has in recent years become the preferred access site for cardiac catheterization around the world.[29,30] Advantages include decreased access-site morbidity, in particular a decrease in major bleeding, and decreased costs. Procedures that may be performed through a transradial approach include cardiac ablation, carotid artery stenting, and renal artery angioplasty; however, access through the radial artery is not without complications, several of which, both common and rare, have been reported.[31] The most common complication is asymptomatic RAO caused by thrombosis, which has a reported incidence of 2% to 18%. The true incidence may be higher, as many of these cases can only be documented through plethysmography and duplex ultrasonography.[29–34]

Acute RAO with distal ischemia is a serious but rare complication. A case of acute hand ischemia following transradial catheterization was encountered in a patient with Raynaud disease who developed persistent spasm of the radial artery, leading to thrombosis.[31] Rhyne and Mann[35]

reported another case requiring radial artery angioplasty for correction of hand ischemia. Such events are rare in patients undergoing transradial catheterization, as patients with an abnormal Allen test are usually directed toward transfemoral catheterization.[36] Radial artery spasm is reported to occur in 5% to 10% of patients during transradial catheterization, and most cases result in no long-term sequelae except for access failure.[33]

Preprocedural risk factors for RAO include female gender, low body mass index, and advanced age.[37] Procedural risk factors for arterial thrombosis include prolonged high-pressure compression of the radial artery to obtain hemostasis following the procedure, repeat entry, and the use of a large introducer sheath.[29–32] Maintaining blood flow through the radial artery while obtaining hemostasis following the procedure has been found to be an important measure to prevent RAO. In a prospective series by Sanmartin and colleagues,[38] the absence of blood flow through the radial artery during the hemostasis process significantly increased the risk of subsequent RAO. Following this study, Pancholy and colleagues[39] performed a randomized comparison to evaluate the efficacy of maintain radial artery patency during the hemostasis process once the catheter is removed. Using a process referred to as patent hemostasis, the investigators applied a compression band to the wrist and then using plethysmography decreased pressure in the band until a plethysmographic waveform was observed on the pulse oximeter, confirming antegrade flow through the radial artery. Patients in this patent hemostasis group had lower rates of RAO than those in the conventional radial artery occlusion group at 24-hour follow-up (5% vs 12%) and after 30 days (1.8% vs 7%). Several devices are now available to perform patent hemostasis, including the TR Band (Terumo Corp, Tokyo, Japan) and the HemoBand (Hemo-Band, Portland, OR, USA) (Fig. 1).[40] The process of patent hemostasis has now become

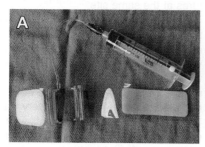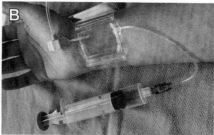

Fig. 1. (A) Example of a compression band for patent hemostasis technique. (B) The band is applied over the radial puncture site and the bladder is then filled with air. Air is released from the bladder until a plethysmographic waveform is observed on the pulse oximeter. The band is left in place for 1 to 2 hours with gradual release of the air in the bladder.

recommended following all transradial catheterization procedures.[33]

Rarer complications following transradial catheterization include arterial perforation, with a reported incidence of 1% or less; this is more common in older and shorter women with tortuous arteries.[41] RAO can also be induced by sheath injury and catheter entrapment (**Fig. 2**).[33] Arterial avulsion and eversion have also been reported.[33,42] Complications such as these can lead to a forearm hematoma and compartment syndrome, necessitating emergent fasciotomy. Other rare complications include the creation of an arterial venous fistula and the development of a radial artery pseudoaneurysm, which can be managed conservatively with compression, percutaneous thrombin injection, use of a TR compression band, or surgical reconstruction.[33,40] In addition to direct arterial injury, other soft-tissue injuries may occur during catheter placement.

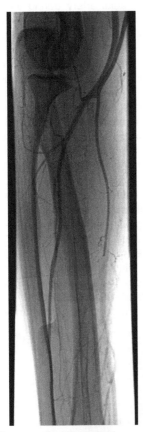

Fig. 2. Angiogram of a 55-year-old man who underwent transradial catheterization. During catheter removal the patient experienced severe pain. Over the next 3 weeks the patient developed symptomatic ischemia of thumb and index finger. The image displays an angiogram of the forearm showing occlusion of radial artery at level of mid forearm.

Median or radial nerve injury can occur with repeated punctures of the radial artery. Complex regional pain syndrome has also been reported.[43,44]

The incidence of many of these complications can be reduced with preventive measures, such as avoidance of multiple punctures at the same site, gentle manipulation of equipment while the catheter is intra-arterial, and careful nonocclusive hemostasis and compression after the procedure.[33] Most importantly, the incidence of RAO has been shown to decrease from 71% to 4.3% in one study with the use of 5000 units of heparin[32] It is now recommended that heparin be given in conjunction with these procedures to maintain radial patency.[32,36] Several best-practice recommendations have been made based on the work of several prospective randomized trials, and have been recently summarized by Caputo and colleagues.[36] These recommendations include: (1) avoiding transradial catheterization in patients with abnormal Allen test or a history of vasospastic disorders (such as Raynaud disease); (2) ensuring adequate administration of heparin during the procedure; and (3) utilization of patent hemostasis techniques following sheath removal.

Indwelling Radial Catheters (Arterial Lines)

It is estimated that 8 million arterial catheters are placed in the United States yearly.[45] Complications following radial artery cannulation with indwelling catheters vary, with a reported incidence of 1% to 35%.[45] Because radial artery catheters stay in place for days, many patients develop complications related to infection and thrombosis. Multiple punctures of the radial artery and repeated cannulation for access have been shown to result in narrowing or occlusion of the radial artery, resulting in access failure and thrombosis.[46] Hence if radial access is deemed necessary, one of the best methods to prevent complications is to avoid repeated arterial punctures at the same site.

Thrombus formation and occlusion of the artery appear to be related to the degree to which the catheter fills the arterial lumen, which may explain why a higher incidence of RAO is seen in women who tend to have a smaller radial arterial diameter.[47] It is now recommended that a 20-gauge catheter be used for radial artery cannulation.[48] The risk for RAO exists in patients with low cardiac output and cannulas left in place longer than 48 to 72 hours.[45,49] As with transradial catheterization, patients who are treated with aspirin or low-dose heparin have a lower incidence of vessel occlusion.[49]

Other conditions that may develop after radial artery cannulation include acute carpal tunnel syndrome.[50] Carpal tunnel syndrome may also develop subacutely, and has been reported 2 weeks after radial arterial cannulation.[51] Cutaneous zygomycosis has been reported in an elderly man with multiple medical problems.[52] Special care needs to be taken in children, as limb shortening resulting from partial arrest of the growth plate has been described following radial artery thrombosis from catheter placement.[53,54] Fortunately, the incidence of permanent ischemic complications is low, with a reported incidence of 0.09% (**Fig. 3**).[55]

The reported incidence of surgical intervention for complications of radial arterial lines is low, and there are few reports in the literature. Unfortunately, the outcomes of surgery are not uniformly successful. Türker and Capdarest-Arest[56] reported a case of persistent hand ischemia despite radial artery reconstruction resulting in hand amputation. A review of patients over a 14-year period at a single center found 30 patients requiring surgery for both infectious complications (such as deep abscesses with or without concomitant arterial thrombosis) and ischemic complications from arterial thrombosis.[57] Valentine and colleagues[58] have reported on 5 patients with acute hand ischemia following radial artery cannulation for arterial monitoring who required surgical intervention. Four of the patients underwent surgery with thrombectomy and patch angioplasty while 1 underwent radial artery reconstruction with an interposition vein graft. Regardless of the patency of the vascular reconstruction, all patients went onto develop gangrene requiring amputation. These studies point to the potential morbidity of RAO.

TREATMENT OF RADIAL ARTERY OCCLUSION

Although asymptomatic RAO does not require intervention, the development of distal ischemia necessitates treatment. If ischemia is detected early, treatment includes conservative and surgical options. Conservative options are probably best for patients with multiple medical comorbidities, and include vasodilators and anticoagulants.[59] Recent publications have suggested that temporary occlusion of the ulnar artery can help in the recanalization of the radial artery. Bernat and colleagues[60] reported that in the cases of acute RAO (as assessed by duplex ultrasonography 3–4 hours after obtaining hemostasis following transradial catheterization), immediate 1-hour ulnar arterial compression was capable of recanalizing occluded radial arteries. Although the mechanism of homolateral ulnar artery compression is not fully understood, this technique offers another nonsurgical treatment option for acute RAO. Homolateral ulnar artery compression in conjunction with systemic heparin therapy is a good first step in the management of symptomatic RAO.

If conservative and medical management are unsuccessful one can consider catheter-directed thrombolytic infusions, which have been reported to be successful in restoring flow through the radial artery and resolving hand ischemia.[61] Thrombolysis of radial arterial occlusion remains controversial, as concerns exist about its effectiveness in forearm and hand thrombosis and the possibility of distal emboli resulting in soft-tissue loss within the hand. Cejna and coleagues[62] reported on 40 patients with acute embolic occlusion of the upper extremity treated with catheter-directed thrombolysis, 28 of whom suffered from isolated embolic events in the forearm and hand. Successful thrombolysis was reported in only 46% of these patients, as opposed to 100% success for those with upper arm occlusions. Cejna's conclusion was that thrombolysis was inferior to surgical intervention for distal thrombosis of the forearm and hand.[62] Angioplasty has also been described in conjunction with catheter-directed thrombolytics for successful management of RAO in the wrist.[63]

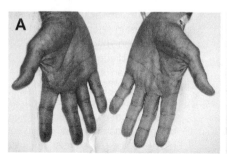
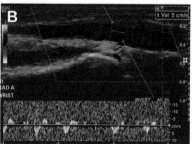

Fig. 3. (*A*) Ischemic discoloration can be seen in the thumb through ring finger of the right hand in this 64-year-old man. Symptomatic ischemia developed following removal of a right radial arterial line. (*B*) Absence of flow in the radial artery was verified by duplex ultrasonography. Reverse TR banding was used to reestablish flow within the radial artery.

Thrombectomy with patch angioplasty or excision of the thrombosed segment followed by reconstruction with vein-graft interposition are the most commonly reported surgical options.[57,58] Despite vascular reconstruction, hand ischemia with a high rate of tissue loss or amputation has been reported. Ongoing hand ischemia may be due to distal embolization from the site of the initial thrombosis, producing areas of distal ischemia that are not treated by radial artery revascularization.[58] In the report by Valentine and colleagues,[58] all patients who underwent arterial reconstruction progressed to tissue loss regardless of the patency of the reconstruction. Reports from other groups have been more promising. In their review of complications from indwelling arterial catheters over a 15-year period, Garg and colleagues[57] found that surgical intervention with thrombectomy and patch angioplasty was successful and able to avoid hand and digit amputations in all cases; however, the overall in-hospital mortality in these patients was 37%, reflecting the underlying comorbidities in this patient population. Recommendations for surgical treatment were for the use of patch angioplasty if surgery was necessary for symptomatic RAO.

For extensive areas of thrombosis or for chronic occlusion, radial artery bypass can be considered. Bypasses for chronic ischemia of the upper extremity have better outcomes than for the lower extremity, with one series reporting a 3-year patency rate of 85% and a limb salvage rate of 100%.[64] Inflow vessels can include the brachial, axillary, and ulnar arteries, whereas outflow targets may include the radial or ulnar artery. In the acute setting thrombectomy and vascular reconstruction is probably a better surgical option, and is certainly less invasive; however, bypass may be the only option for chronic ischemia that develops after radial artery harvest.

SUMMARY

Complications after radial artery harvest and arterial cannulation are rare, but can potentially be catastrophic. As transradial catheterization becomes more popular, the hand surgeon will increasingly be called upon to evaluate patients with acute and chronic ischemic complications. Prevention is the best means of avoiding RAO. Preoperative screening can identify patients at risk of ischemia before radial artery cannulation, and these patients should be diverted to other access sites for catheterization procedures. The use of anticoagulation and nonocclusive hemostasis may decrease the incidence of acute RAO. Heightening physicians' awareness of the complications is the best means of improving patients' outcomes.

REFERENCES

1. Piccolo R, Galasso G, Capuano E, et al. Transradial versus transfemoral approach in patients undergoing percutaneous coronary intervention for acute coronary syndrome. A meta-analysis and trial sequential analysis of randomized controlled trials. PLoS One 2014;9:e96127.
2. Coleman SS, Anson BJ. Arterial patterns in the hand based upon a study of 650 specimens. Surg Gynecol Obstet 1961;113:409–24.
3. Riekkinen HV, Karkola KO, Kankainen A. The radial artery is larger than the ulnar. Ann Thorac Surg 2003;75:882–4.
4. Loh YJ, Nakao M, Tan WD, et al. Factors influencing radial artery size. Asian Cardiovasc Thorac Ann 2007;15:324–6.
5. Ashraf T, Panhwar Z, Habib S, et al. Size of radial and ulnar artery in local population. J Pak Med Assoc 2010;60:817–9.
6. Barbeau GR, Arsenault F, Dugas L, et al. Evaluation of the ulnopalmar arterial arches with pulse oximetry and plethysmography: comparison with the Allen's test in 1010 patients. Am Heart J 2004; 147(3):489–93.
7. Higgins JP. A reassessment of the role of the radial forearm flap in upper extremity reconstruction. J Hand Surg 2011;36A:1237–40.
8. Kohonen M, Teerenhovi O, Terho T, et al. Is the Allen test reliable enough? Eur J Cardiothorac Surg 2007;32:902–5.
9. Stead SW, Stirt JA. Assessment of digital blood flow and palmar collateral circulation. Allen's test vs. photoplethysmography. Int J Clin Monit Comput 1985;2:29–34.
10. Starnes SL, Wolk SW, Lampman RM, et al. Noninvasive evaluation of hand circulation before radial artery harvest for coronary artery bypass grafting. J Thorac Cardiovasc Surg 1999;117:261–6.
11. Jarvis MA, Jarvis CL, Jones PR, et al. Reliability of Allen's test in selection of patients for radial artery harvest. Ann Thorac Surg 2000;70:1362–5.
12. Rodriguez-Niedenfuhr M, Sanudo JR, Vazquez T, et al. Median artery revisited. J Anat 1999;199: 57–63.
13. Greenwood MJ, Della-Siega AJ, Fretz EB, et al. Vascular communications of the hand in patients being considered for transradial coronary angiography: is the Allen's test accurate? J Am Coll Cardiol 2005;46(11):2013–7.
14. Jones BM, O'Brien CJ. Acute ischaemia of the hand resulting from elevation of a radial forearm flap. Br J Plast Surg 1985;38(3):396–7.

15. Varley I, Carter LM, Wales CJ, et al. Ischaemia of the hand after harvest of a radial forearm flap. Br J Oral Maxillofac Surg 2008;46(5):403–5.

16. Talegon-Melendez A, Ciria-Llorens G, Gomez-Cia T, et al. Elevating the radial forearm flap: prospective study using color duplex imaging. J Ultrasound Med 1999;18:553–8.

17. Royse AG, Royse CF, Maleskar A, et al. Harvest of the radial artery for coronary artery surgery preserves maximal blood flow of the forearm. Ann Thorac Surg 2004;78:539–42.

18. Dumanian GA, Segalman K, Mispireta LA, et al. Radial artery use in bypass grafting does not change digital blood flow or hand function. Ann Thorac Surg 1998;65:1284–7.

19. Meland NB, Core GB, Hoverman VR. The radial forearm flap donor site: should we vein graft the artery? A comparative study. Plast Reconstr Surg 1993;91(5):865–70.

20. Manabe S, Tabuchi N, Toyama M, et al. Oxygen pressure measurement during grip exercise reveals exercise intolerance after radial harvest. Ann Thorac Surg 2004;77:2066–70.

21. Gaudino M, Serricchio M, Tondi P, et al. Chronic compensatory increase in ulnar flow and accelerated atherosclerosis after radial artery removal for coronary artery bypass. J Thorac Cardiovasc Surg 2005;130:9–12.

22. Gaudino M, Glieca F, Luciani N, et al. Ten-year echo-Doppler evaluation of forearm circulation following radial artery removal for coronary artery bypass grafting. Eur J Cardiothorac Surg 2006;29:71–3.

23. Gaudino M, Anselmi A, Serricchio M, et al. Late haemodynamic and functional consequences of radial artery removal on the forearm circulation. Int J Cardiol 2008;129:255–8.

24. Lee HS, Chang BC, Heo YJ. Digital blood flow after radial artery harvest for coronary artery bypass grafting. Ann Thorac Surg 2004;77:2071–4.

25. Lee HS, Heo YJ, Chang BC. Long term digital blood flow after radial artery harvesting for coronary artery bypass grafting. Eur J Cardiothorac Surg 2005;27:99–103.

26. Royse AG, Chang GS, Nicholas DM, et al. No late ulnar artery atheroma after radial artery harvest for coronary artery bypass surgery. Ann Thorac Surg 2008;85:891–4.

27. Schena S, Crabtree TD, Baker KA, et al. Absence of deterioration of vascular function of the donor limb at late follow-up after radial artery harvesting. J Thorac Cardiovasc Surg 2011;142:298–301.

28. Higgins JP, Orlando GS, Chang P, et al. Hypothenar hammer syndrome after radial forearm flap harvest: a case report. J Hand Surg 2001;26A:772–5.

29. Turner S, Sacrinty M, Manogue M, et al. Transitioning to the radial artery as the preferred access site for cardiac catheterization: an academic medical center experience. Catheter Cardiovasc Interv 2012;80:247–57.

30. Applegate R, Sacrinty M, Schafer P, et al. Cost effectiveness of radial access for diagnostic cardiac catheterization and coronary intervention. Catheter Cardiovasc Interv 2013;82:E375–84.

31. Kanei Y, Kwan T, Nakra NC. Transradial cardiac catheterization: a review of access site complications. Catheter Cardiovasc Interv 2011;78:840–6.

32. Spaulding C, Lefevre T, Funck F, et al. Left radial approach for coronary angiography: results of a prospective study. Catheter Cardiovasc Interv 1996;39:365–70.

33. Dandekar VK, Vidovich MI, Shroff AR. Complications of transradial catheterization. Cardiovasc Revasc Med 2012;13(1):39–50.

34. Brancati MF, Burzotta F, Coluccia V, et al. The occurrence of radial artery occlusion following catheterization. Expert Rev Cardiovasc Ther 2012;10(10):1287–95.

35. Rhyne D, Mann T. Hand ischemia resulting from a transradial intervention: successful management with radial artery angioplasty. Catheter Cardiovasc Interv 2010;76(3):383–6.

36. Caputo RP, Tremmel JA, Rao S, et al. Transradial arterial access for coronary and peripheral procedures: executive summary by the Transradial Committee of the SCAI. Catheter Cardiovasc Interv 2011;78(6):823–39.

37. Calvino-Santos RA, Vasquez-Rodriguez JM, Salgado-Fernandez J, et al. Management of iatrogenic radial artery perforation. Catheter Cardiovasc Interv 2004;61:74–8.

38. Sanmartin M, Gomez M, Rumoroso JR, et al. Interruption of blood flow during compression and radial artery occlusion after transradial catheterization. Catheter Cardiovasc Interv 2007;70(2):185–9.

39. Pancholy S, Coppola J, Patel T, et al. Prevention of radial artery occlusion—patent hemostasis evaluation trial (PROPHET study): a randomized comparison of traditional versus patency documented hemostasis after transradial catheterization. Catheter Cardiovasc Interv 2008;72(3):335–40.

40. Pancholy SB. Impact of two different hemostatic devices on radial artery outcomes after transradial catheterization. J Invasive Cardiol 2009;21(3):101–4.

41. Alkhouli M, Cohen HA, Bashir R. Radial artery avulsion—a rare complication of transradial catheterization. Catheter Cardiovasc Interv 2014. [Epub ahead of print].

42. Liou M, Tung F, Kanei Y, et al. Treatment of radial artery pseudoaneurysm using a novel compression device. J Invasive Cardiol 2010;22:293–5.

43. Papadimos TJ, Hofmann JP. Radial artery thrombosis, palmar arch systolic blood velocities, and

chronic regional pain syndrome 1 following transradial cardiac catheterization. Catheter Cardiovasc Interv 2002;57:537–40.

44. Sasano N, Tsuda T, Sasno H, et al. A case of complex regional pain syndrome type II after transradial coronary intervention. J Anesth 2004;18:310–2.

45. Scheer B, Perel A, Pfeiffer UJ. Clinical review: complications and risk factors of peripheral arterial catheters used for haemodynamic monitoring in anaesthesia and intensive care medicine. Crit Care 2002;6(3):199–204.

46. Sakai H, Ikeda S, Harada T, et al. Limitations of successive transradial approach in the same arm: the Japanese experience. Catheter Cardiovasc Interv 2001;54:204–8.

47. Bedford RF. Wrist circumference predicts the risk of radial-arterial occlusion after cannulation. Anesthesiology 1978;48:377–8.

48. Davis FM. Radial artery cannulation: influence of catheter size and material on arterial occlusion. Anaesth Intensive Care 1978;6:49–53.

49. Davis FM, Stewart JM. Radial artery cannulation: a prospective study in patients undergoing cardiothoracic surgery. Br J Anaesth 1980;52:41–7.

50. Martin SD, Sharrock NE, Mineo R, et al. Acute exacerbation of carpal tunnel syndrome after radial artery cannulation. J Hand Surg Am 1993;18:455–8.

51. Sanchez-Garcia ML, Riesgo MJ, Benito-Alcala MC, et al. Late ischemia and carpal tunnel syndrome secondary to catheterization of the radial artery. Rev Esp Anestesiol Reanim 1997;44:201–3.

52. Kapadia S, Polenakovik H. Cutaneous zygomycosis following attempted radial artery cannulation. Skinmed 2004;3:336–8.

53. Guy RL, Holland JP, Shaw DG, et al. Limb shortening secondary to complications of vascular cannulae in the neonatal period. Skeletal Radiol 1990;19:423–5.

54. Macnicol MF, Anagnostopoulos J. Arrest of the growth plate after arterial cannulation in infancy. J Bone Joint Surg Br 2000;2:172–5.

55. Brzezinski M, Luisetti T, London MJ. Radial artery cannulation: a comprehensive review of recent anatomic and physiologic investigations. Anesth Analg 2009;109:1763–81.

56. Türker T, Capdarest-Arest N. Acute hand ischemia after radial artery cannulation resulting in amputation. Chir Main 2014;33(4):299–302. http://dx.doi.org/10.1016/j.main.2014.05.001.

57. Garg K, Howell BW, Saltzberg SS, et al. Open surgical management of complications from indwelling radial artery catheters. J Vasc Surg 2013;58:1325–30.

58. Valentine RJ, Modrall JG, Clagett GP. Hand ischemia after radial artery cannulation. J Am Coll Surg 2005;201:18–22.

59. Zankl AR, Andrassy M, Volz C, et al. Radial artery thrombosis following transradial coronary angiography: incidence and rationale for treatment of symptomatic patients with low-molecular-weight heparins. Clin Res Cardiol 2010;99:841–7.

60. Bernat I, Bertrand OF, Rokyta R, et al. Efficacy and safety of transient ulnar artery compression to recanalize acute radial artery occlusion after transradial catheterization. Am J Cardiol 2011;107(11):1698–701.

61. Geschwind JF, Dagli MS, Lambert DL, et al. Thrombolytic therapy in the setting of arterial line-induced ischemia. J Endovasc Ther 2003;10:590–4.

62. Cejna M, Salomonowitz E, Wohlschlager H, et al. rt-PA thrombolysis in acute thromboembolic upper-extremity arterial occlusion. Cardiovasc Intervent Radiol 2001;24(4):218–23.

63. Pasha AK, Elder MD, Malik UE, et al. Symptomatic radial artery thrombosis successfully treated with endovascular approach via femoral access route. Cardiovasc Revasc Med 2014. pii:S1553-8389(14)00127-4. [Epub ahead of print].

64. Hughes K, Hamdan A, Schermerhorn M, et al. Bypass for chronic ischemia of the upper extremity: results in 20 patients. J Vasc Surg 2007;46:303–7.

Role and Rationale for Extended Periarterial Sympathectomy in the Management of Severe Raynaud Syndrome
Techniques and Results

Wyndell H. Merritt, MD[a,b],*

KEYWORDS

- Raynaud syndrome • Extended periarterial sympathectomy • Botulinum toxin
- Evidence-based data

KEY POINTS

- Experimental studies of periarterial sympathectomy demonstrate a profound adrenergic effect only at the site of adventitial stripping, with limited decrease of vasoconstriction distally and no decrease in vasoconstriction of the proximal vasculature; this is likely due to the anatomic arrangement of segmental sympathetic branching from the adjacent nerves directly to the vessels.
- Patients with connective tissue disease will likely later develop occlusions proximal to sites of palmar and finger periarterial sympathectomy, and can be protected by extended periarterial sympathectomy, which includes adventitial stripping of the ulnar artery in the distal forearm and the dorsal radial artery in the snuffbox region.
- In patients with connective tissue disease who have ulnar artery occlusion, vein-graft reconstruction can usually be accomplished by the end-to-side technique to the superficial vascular arch and proximal ulnar artery, leaving collaterals intact, and the donor veins are found in the forearm. In this group of patients vascular reconstruction should be accompanied by extended periarterial sympathectomy.
- At surgery, topical botulinum toxin (Botox) applied to the exposed arteries and vein grafts affords prolonged vasodilatation, and Botox injections of the unoperated hand at that time will allow bilateral relief from ischemic discomfort.
- Extended periarterial sympathectomy may offer prolonged improvement by reducing the frequency and severity of ischemic Raynaud attacks, and decreasing recurrence of ischemic ulcerations; the mechanism may be by reducing vascular change induced by reperfusion injury following frequent severe Raynaud attacks.

 Videos of common volar artery branching into proper digital vessels to the right, superficial vascular arch branching into common volar arteries, and an ulnar artery as it becomes the superficial arch accompany this article at http://www.hand.theclinics.com/

The author has nothing to disclose.
[a] Division of Plastic & Reconstructive Surgery, Virginia Commonwealth University, 830 East Main Street, Richmond, VA 23298, USA; [b] Department of Plastic & Maxillofacial Surgery, University of Virginia, 1215 Lee Street, Charlottesville, VA 22903, USA
* 7660 East Parham Road, Suite 200, Henrico, VA 23294.
E-mail address: wyndell@hotmail.com

INTRODUCTION

On comprendra sans peine, jel'espere, qu'en presence d'une maladie dont tant de points sont encore obscures, je ne sois pas en mesure de formuler un traitement complet a lui opposer. [I hope it will be readily understood that for a disease so many aspects of which are still obscure, I cannot formulate a complete treatment.]

—M. Raynaud, 1862[1]

More than 150 years after Raynaud's description of this disorder, his disclaimer remains valid. Severe Raynaud syndrome remains a controversial unsolved problem because of our inability to "formulate a complete treatment" that is universally successful, and because "so many aspects…are still obscure." This problem is especially true of patients with connective tissue disease who all too often present to the hand surgeon weeks or months after digital necrosis or gangrenous changes, having suffered unremitting ischemic pain. In the past, simple amputations of gangrenous fingertips led to reoperation more proximally because of ischemic change in the amputation stump. Furthermore, adjacent digits developed similar change, requiring further amputations (**Fig. 1**). Many articles on Raynaud syndrome are pessimistic about any long-term benefit from surgery, other than debridement and digital amputation.[2–5] Much of this pessimism derives from poor results reported in cervicothoracic sympathectomy when done in patients with connective tissue disease.[6] After Flatt's[7] 1980 contribution describing successful distal digital artery periarterial sympathectomy for Raynaud syndrome in 8 patients (mostly frostbite but including 2 with connective tissue disease[7]), the value of this operation for patients with connective tissue

disease became an important question. There is much debate and little consensus regarding surgical indications (palliative or beneficial), surgical technique (extent of dissection), or even if the procedure is worthwhile at all; however, among the relatively small number of reports available, results of distal microvascular adventectomy seem encouraging, although somewhat variable.

At present, most clinicians still regard surgery for Raynaud syndrome as a salvage procedure for gangrenous change after failed pharmacologic management. Over the past 33 years this author has dealt with more than 100 of these difficult patients, which has led to significant alteration in surgical indications, preoperative evaluation, surgical technique, and attitude about the procedure from one of palliation to a belief that there can be a sustained benefit. Because the patient with connective tissue disease represents the most severe of the digital artery sympathectomy surgical candidates, this article emphasizes procedures for this group of patients, including experience with mixed connective tissue disease (55% of the series), scleroderma (38%) and lupus (4%), evolving into a surgical approach the author describes as "extended periarterial sympathectomy" that is not appropriate for other causes of Raynaud syndrome, such as frostbite, trauma, or hypothenar hammer syndrome. An effort is made to explain the rationale and results of the current surgical approach of the author's team (referred to subjectively throughout this article) regarding this specific group of patients.

THE CONUNDRUM OF EVIDENCE-BASED DATA IN RAYNAUD SYNDROME

Clinical syndromes often suffer from lack of objective standardized diagnostic criteria, and Raynaud syndrome is no exception. Initial criteria by Maurice Raynaud included the characteristic triad of digital skin vasospastic color change in response to cold exposure or emotional stress. This triad is no longer considered essential for diagnosis, although it occurs in two-thirds of patients. Precise objective criteria for diagnosis are not agreed upon, with many investigators who believe a carefully documented history is the best criterion, and a simple questionnaire the best tool for diagnosis. Furthermore, measurement parameters for study results are equally variable, with some reporting the incidence and severity of Raynaud attacks, and others the healing of ulceration and amputation stumps or changes in cold recovery testing. Under such circumstances, each investigator determines one's own parameters for diagnosis and outcome measurements, and no meaningful

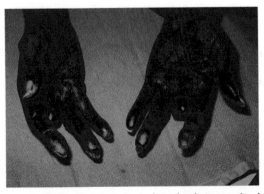

Fig. 1. Medical management alone leads to proximal amputations and progression to ischemic necrosis in adjacent digits.

comparisons can be made for evidence-based conclusions among the various reports.

Although all Raynaud syndrome reports suffer these limitations, surgical management is especially difficult to study because patients are typically referred with an ischemic crisis after medical management failure from variable precipitating causes, and, as such, they are not amenable to randomization given the differing etiology. Instead, they need individualized management for the particular circumstance, using the best clinical experience and common sense available.

For example, an ischemic ulcerated digit in a patient with Buerger disease may be cured by botulinum toxin (Botox) injection if the patient stops smoking, whereas the scleroderma patient with gangrenous digits and an occluded ulnar artery may need vein-graft reconstruction and extended periarterial sympathectomy with topical arterial Botox to heal amputation stumps and avoid further progressive digit loss. Meanwhile, the Raynaud patient with hypothenar hammer syndrome needs only resection and replacement of the occluded ulnar artery segment with a vein or arterial graft for cure.

Furthermore, there is no agreement among surgeons regarding which vessels and how much adventitia to strip, with variation from only 3 to 4 mm per vessel[7] to an extensive amount from forearm to fingers (**Table 1**).[8]

Attempts to pool these reports cannot provide meaningful data because of the variable techniques, variable indications, variable etiologic factors, variable diagnostic criteria, and variable result parameters. As clinicians our best hope at present is to extrapolate animal studies and resort to common sense and clinical experience until we can better agree on diagnostic criteria, treatment result measurements, and standardized procedures to meet the higher levels for evidence-based data.

PATHOPHYSIOLOGY OF RAYNAUD SYNDROME

In 1862 Maurice Raynaud described vasospasm causing the triad of fingertip color change, classically described as Raynaud syndrome:

- White (pallor)
- Blue (cyanosis)
- Red (hyperemia)

This triad is often followed by pain, numbness, and sometimes digital gangrene (**Fig. 2**). Now, 152 years later, we still cannot explain the biological mechanisms for these dramatic changes, nor any consistently successful method of management.

There is a puzzling spectrum of more than 40 precipitating or associated factors that are widely varied,[8] including: anatomic factors such as thoracic outlet syndrome, dialysis shunting, and obstructive arteriosclerotic disease; injuries such as vibratory (white finger syndrome) and frostbite; toxic drugs such as nicotine, lead, vinyl chloride, and β-blocking antihypertensive medications; diseases such as scleroderma (95% incidence), lupus (91%), dermatomyositis (30%), rheumatoid

Table 1
Technical differences in digital artery sympathectomy: how much does one strip?

Digital Artery and Amount Stripped	Authors,[Ref.] Year
Common volar bifurcation into proper digital arteries, 3–5 mm	Flatt,[7] 1980
Common volar plus proper digital arteries, 5–10 mm	Egloff et al,[61] 1982
Common volar plus proper digital arteries, 20 mm	Wilgis,[55] 1981; Morgan,[75] 1991
Common volar from arch plus proper digital arteries	Levine et al,[65] 1984; Zachary et al,[56] 1995
Common volar plus entire arch and proper digital arteries	Jones et al,[66,68] 1987
Segments of radial and ulnar vessels plus common volar and proper digital arteries	El-Gammal & Blair,[62] 1991
Ulnar and radial arteries at wrist (2 cm), radial artery at snuffbox plus superficial arch and take-off of common volar vessels	Koman et al,[57] 2005
Ulnar artery at wrist to entire arch, common volar and proper digital vessels into the fingers	O'Brien et al,[42] 1992
Ulnar artery distal one-third forearm including nerve of Henle, wrist and entire arch, common volar and proper digital vessels into web, sometimes to the level of proximal interphalangeal joint; dorsal radial artery, plus topical Botox	Merritt,[8,76] 1997, 2007

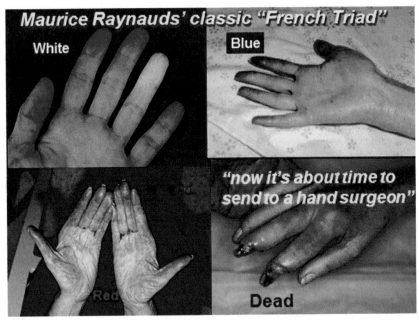

Fig. 2. Raynaud's original 1862 description was of blanched, cyanotic, then erythematous coloration, the "French triad," which could then lead to necrosis.

arthritis (11%), cancer, and hypothyroidism; and rheologic causes such as cryoglobulinemia and polycythemia vera. However, the largest group of patients described as having Raynaud disease or primary Raynaud syndrome has no known associated factors at all, other than being 10 times more common in women.

That such different disorders are united by similar manifestations attracts a search for a single systemic or local factor, but no such factor is yet held accountable. The 2 most widely debated theories are whether the syndrome represents (1) central changes causing hyperactivity of the sympathetic nervous system as believed by Raynaud in 1862,[1] or (2) local vessel changes at the periphery as believed by Lewis in 1926.[9] After 88 years of debate, a unifying hypothesis is needed. Raynaud observed vasospastic attacks precipitated by both emotional and cold stress, leading him to reason that increased central nervous system sympathetic activity must be the explanation. Indeed, emotional stress is currently reported in one-third of patients with characteristic attacks.[3,10] However, evidence that local factors might be more important than the central nervous system includes experiments using skin microelectrodes that do not measure any increased activity in sympathetic outflow, only altered response to cold stimuli,[11] and measurement of circulating catecholamines showing no increase over normal levels in Raynaud patients.[12] Although there are findings suggesting

altered responsiveness of α- and β-blocking receptors to catecholamines, isolation of any specific responsible endothelial factor has not been achieved, even though obvious pathologic change in distal vessels is well documented.

Central Neuropeptide Dysregulation

In 1995 Kahaleh and Matucci-Cerinic[13] proposed a provocative hypothesis suggesting that dysregulation of the central neuropeptide system could provide the mechanism for Raynaud attacks. This concept is attractive because it reconciles studies that show both central and peripheral mechanisms to be present. A powerful neurologic influence on both vasodilatation and vasoconstriction can be mediated by the release of neuropeptides present in the sensory nervous system (substance P [SP] and calcitonin gene-related peptide [CGRP]), sympathetic nervous system (neuropeptide Y [NPY] and norepinephrine), and parasympathetic nervous system (vasoactive intestinal peptide [VIP] and acetylcholine). Some are vasoconstrictors (NPY) and some are vasodilators (CGRP, SP, and VIP), and their action may be endothelial-dependent (SP) or they may act directly on the smooth muscle cell (CGRP, NPY, VIP).

These neuropeptides are known to be synthesized in the mid-brain and spinal cord, where some mediate pain perception but also may be secreted at peripheral nerve endings, such as afferent pain endings and sympathetic endings, where they cause several vasoactive and inflammatory responses.[14] Regulation of this neuropeptide system is poorly understood, but it is known that temperature alteration may induce their secretion and that sensory neuropeptides are found in abundance in human digital skin.[15] In support of this hypothesis, Bunker and colleagues[16] demonstrated that direct infusion of the neuropeptide CGRP (a potent vasodilator) reverses vasospasm in Raynaud attacks, and is reported to promote healing of ischemic ulceration. The facts that Raynaud patients have frequent placebo response, transcutaneous electrical nerve stimulation (TENS) unit and temperature biofeedback response, and vasospastic episodes in response to emotional stress certainly implies the presence of centrally mediated mechanisms, whereas distal obvious anatomic vascular change and failure of sympathetic blocks and proximal sympathectomy along with favorable response to distal Botox injections implies a peripheral origin. Dysregulation of the neuropeptide system causing repeated Raynaud attacks with subsequent vascular alteration caused by reperfusion injury could explain the presence of both central and peripheral factors, and the peculiar tricolor sequence of vascular response known as the French triad, with differing neuropeptides having profound opposing vasoactive responses in sequence: white, blue, and red. Raynaud syndrome certainly occurs at anatomic sites where there are the highest numbers of arteriovenous anastomoses that control thermal regulation and capillary blood flow, and also dense concentration of afferent nociceptor sensory nerve endings, such as fingertips, toes, tongue tip, pinnae of the ears, and tip of the nose, with symptoms having been reported in all of these sites.

Reperfusion Injury

It is of interest that patients with scleroderma typically give a history of Raynaud attacks an average of 11.5 years before positive laboratory diagnosis.[17] Because these Raynaud attacks may be a symptom of occult connective tissue disease for such a long interval, Blunt and Porter[18] suggest the terms Raynaud disease and Raynaud phenomenon be abandoned, using only the term Raynaud syndrome for all patients. Pathologic study of postmortem scleroderma patients show digital artery intimal fibrosis and thickening, with the lumen narrowed to less than one-fourth of its diameter in 79%[19] and ulnar artery thickening to an extent that may completely occlude this vessel in almost 50%, which is the principal blood supply

of the hand. It is conceivable that the dysregulated neuropeptide system may be the primary mechanism, suggesting that the intimal fibrosis and thickening may actually be the result of frequent and severe Raynaud attacks attributable to reperfusion injury to the vessel walls from the ischemia and reperfusion cycles.[13] In other words, the vascular anatomic changes may be the result rather than the cause of Raynaud attacks, but as the vessel wall thickens and narrows the attacks will become increasingly severe. If so, early control of vasospastic attacks by either pharmacologic or by extensive microvascular perivascular sympathectomy conceivably could prevent some of these changes.

NONSURGICAL MANAGEMENT
Hand Therapy

There is no cure for patients with Raynaud phenomenon associated with connective tissue disease.[2,20] Hand therapy and pharmacologic and surgical management should be coordinated, with surgery postponed until other measures fail. Not infrequently, patients present to the surgeon without comprehensive medical management, and rarely have they ever been seen by a hand therapist. Patients need to be taught preventive measures that can reduce attacks, such as avoiding cold exposure, cigarette smoking, caffeinated beverages, vibratory exposure, and vasoconstrictive drugs such as most decongestants, β-adrenergic antihypertensive medication, amphetamines, and cocaine. Biofeedback therapy,[21] "induced vasodilatation,"[22] and specific exercise therapy[23] are successful hand therapy measures in some patients who have not developed ischemic ulcerations, and the hand therapist is an invaluable partner in monitoring and encouraging these patients. Other measures, such as acupuncture,[24] TENS,[25] stellate ganglion block,[26] and spinal cord stimulation[27] are of less convincing value in patients with connective disease.

Pharmacologic Management

Pharmacologic management is the principal treatment for Raynaud syndrome, but is reported to benefit only 40% to 66% of patients, and rarely ever offers complete relief.[28–30] The US Food and Drug Administration has approved no single pharmacologic agent as safe and effective for Raynaud syndrome, although several are classified as "possibly effective."[31] Most of the Raynaud syndrome literature is devoted to controversy over which medicines are most effective, with choices varying from medications designed to vasodilate, such as intravenous CGRP, or prevent vasoconstriction, such as calcium-channel blockers, α-adrenergic blockers, angiotensin-converting enzyme inhibitors, and serotonin receptor antagonists; drugs that alter prostaglandin metabolism such as prostaglandin E1, and drugs that have a rheologic effect, such as aspirin and pentoxifylline. The most effective and widely accepted medications are the calcium-channel blockers (especially nifedipine, diltiazem, and amlodipine besylate), and aspirin. Parenteral infusion of prostaglandin E1 will reverse a crisis situation, but if used for more than 3 days will cause generalized edema.[8] CGRP will also reverse vasospasm, but is available only experimentally at present.

Botulinum Toxin

Botox will paralyze smooth muscle, and injection along the vasculature has proved a recent rewarding addition for patients having vasospastic crisis. In surgical patients with bilateral difficulty we use injections in the unoperated hand at the time of surgery with pronounced relief, as well as for patients with an ischemic pain crisis (**Fig. 3**). When effective, this produces relief from vasospastic pain soon after injection, and has resulted in healed ulcerations.[32,33] Neumeister and colleagues[34] measured a 300% increased laser Doppler perfusion immediately after injection. Unfortunately, Medicare and many insurance health management organizations still do not approve this simple measure, regarding it as "experimental," although alternatives are far more expensive and morbid. In our experience, most patients redevelop symptoms approximately 3 to 6 months following Botox injection, and we have regarded it as an adjunctive measure in patients with severe disease. It is particularly useful to cure Buerger disease without surgery if the patient will stop smoking. Connective tissue disease patients with an occluded ulnar artery are less likely to obtain adequate relief from Botox alone, although in the absence of frank gangrene it should be attempted whenever insurance authorization can be obtained.

Fat Grafting

Grafting approximately 30cc of fat to hands of Raynaud's patients is reported as providing significant subjective improvement in pain, recurrent ulceration and reduction of Raynaud's attacks in 80% of 13 patients.[35] The presumed benefit was by stem cells within the fat grafts, producing angiogenesis as had been reported in murine radiated model.[36] Objective parameters were equivocal in the 18-month follow-up, but this remains a provocative arena for investigation.

PREOPERATIVE PATIENT EVALUATION

Objective diagnostic criteria for Raynaud syndrome are not agreed upon, with history and questionnaires used by most investigators.[37] The characteristic French-tricolor vascular change is no longer considered essential for diagnosis, although it occurs in two-thirds of the patients.

Cold Recovery Testing

If the diagnosis is in question, our hand therapists use cold recovery time as the primary diagnostic tool, placing digits in a water bath at 20°C for 1 minute, with a positive diagnosis when there is no recovery of baseline temperature measurement after 20 minutes or longer. This method was introduced by Porter and colleagues,[38] who found that control subjects recovered within 5 to 20 minutes (averaging 10 minutes). However, we do not use cold exposure in patients whose diagnosis is obvious, especially if they have ischemic change and are at risk of harm. This cold recovery test lacks specificity, in that heavy smokers with no characteristics of Raynaud syndrome frequently cannot pass the test.

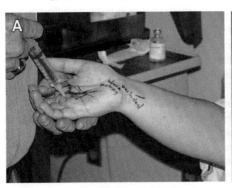
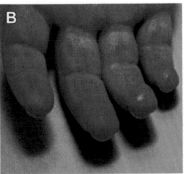

Fig. 3. (*A*) Scleroderma patient with cyanosis and ischemic pain of the ring digit, relieved by Botox injection (100 units) for 4 months. (*B*) The patient chose to have successful sympathectomy and ulnar artery vein graft after recurrence.

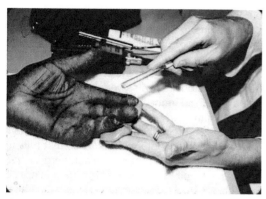

Fig. 4. Semmes-Weinstein monofilament measurement testing preoperatively.

Semmes-Weinstein Monofilament Testing

Sensory testing is of particular help in these patients. Raynaud patients have significantly greater loss of sensation compared with controls following cold exposure,[39] and patients with severe difficulty will have decreased Semmes-Weinstein monofilament measurements, often with the unusual finding of better sensation in the palm and base of their digits than distally (**Fig. 4**). This measurement is useful to verify improvement following periarterial sympathectomy, in that we expect severely afflicted digits to regain improved sensibility after surgery.

Allen and Doppler Testing

The Allen test should be done because of frequent ulnar artery occlusion, especially in scleroderma patients. Doppler ultrasonographic mapping of vessels is of enormous value in assessing all patients with Raynaud syndrome, especially those for surgical consideration.[8] Particular attention should be paid to the ulnar artery at the distal forearm and wrist, superficial vascular arch in the palm and dorsal radial artery, and the common volar and proper digital vessels. However, patent common volar and proper digital arteries are often not audible in the office setting, but may be easily heard in the operating room after the vasodilatation induced by general or block anesthesia. Laser Doppler study has been reassuring in the immediate postoperative setting, with improvement generally measured at 50% to 300%,[8] but has not been essential for management, and seems somewhat variable in our experience.

Radiologic Testing

Radiologic evaluation is valuable in surgical candidates, especially if there is any clinical evidence of proximal occlusion. Although arteriography is regarded as the gold standard for evaluation,[40] it has not been as accurate as magnetic resonance (MR) angiography in our experience for patients with connective tissue disease.[41] Arteriography has caused vasospasm that made the ulnar artery and superficial vascular arch appear occluded, which we later found to be patent at surgery. This feature was also observed by O'Brien and colleagues,[42] and may be due to radiopaque contrast media, which has been shown experimentally to cause arteriolar spasm.[43] Furthermore, patients with mixed connective tissue disease, lupus, or scleroderma are already at greater risk for renal problems, which can also be a complication of allergy to radiographic dye.

MR angiography imaging is a noninvasive reliable alternative to conventional angiography of the hand and wrist[41] with the advantages of oblique, cross-sectional, and longitudinal views of the fingers and hands, lower morbidity, and less expense than conventional angiography. It requires a radiologist with appropriate equipment and degree of interest to obtain all of the planes of measurement needed (**Fig. 5**).

Unfortunately, at present Medicare and some commercial insurance organizations may refuse to approve vascular evaluation with MR angiography in the upper extremity, even though it seems safer, more accurate in patients with connective tissue disease, and a cheaper evaluation technique.

Radiographic dye angiography or computed tomographic angiography is preferred for patients with Raynaud syndrome who do not have connective tissue disease, such as ulnar artery hypothenar hammer syndrome, atherosclerotic disease, occlusion from emboli, or thoracic outlet syndrome, because arteriographic dye assessment provides a better evaluation of the intravascular anatomy.

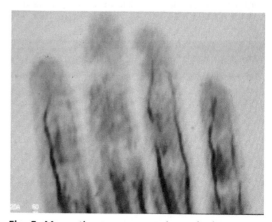

Fig. 5. Magnetic resonance angiography better outlines flow in smaller vessels than radiographic dye angiography.

Functional Assessment of the Hand

A careful preoperative functional assessment of the hand should be done on all patients with Raynaud syndrome, including measurement of sensation, manual dexterity, range of motion, strength, baseline temperature, and skin and digit appearance, because many of these patients have or will develop sclerodactyly changes that need to be monitored.

RATIONALE FOR PERIARTERIAL SYMPATHECTOMY

Arterial smooth muscle has only one function, vasoconstriction. The concept of direct sympathetic denervation of arterial muscle to reduce vasoconstriction is by no means new, having been first suggested by Leriche and later performed by Jabollet in 1899 on axillary vessels of Raynaud patients.[44] Leriche reported its value on the femoral artery in 1913. However, it was not until 1980 that Flatt[7] introduced the concept of distal vessel periarterial sympathectomy. Based on Pick's[45] classic text on the autonomic nervous system, Flatt reasoned that proximal cervicothoracic sympathectomy failure could be caused by alternative pathways to the brachial plexus from the sinovertebral nerve, the carotid plexus, and the nerve of Koontz. Contributions to the sympathetic supply in the hand is directly from the peripheral nerves with multiple segmental branches to the adjacent vessels in the forearm, wrist, palm, and fingers; for example, digital nerves have multiple segmental sympathetic branches to the corresponding digital arteries (**Fig. 6**), and the distal ulnar artery in the forearm is supplied by the ulnar nerve, usually with a specific branch, the nerve of Henle, in addition to multiple smaller segmental branches.[46,47] Pick's descriptions and our clinical observations show the sympathetic contributions to be particularly intense at sites of bifurcation, such as where the superficial arch branches into the common volar vessels, and then their bifurcation into the proper digital vessels (**Fig. 7**). Mitchell[48] observed that sympathetic fibers arborized in the adventitia of these vessels, and Morgan and colleagues[49] confirmed that these fibers are confined to the adventitia without deeper penetration into the media, so that adventitial stripping should remove the adrenergic nerve endings. Rabbit ear experiments demonstrated that there was no sympathetic reinnervation after a year following periarterial stripping of vessels.[50]

Soon after World War I, Leriche and Jabollet's periarterial sympathectomy concept became controversial because of the anatomic fact that there is little evidence of long centripetal sympathetic nerves running along the arteries; rather, it is recognized there are multiple segmental sympathetic branches innervating arteries proximal and distal to the sites of perivascular sympathectomy. It was recommended that proximal cervicothoracic sympathectomy seemed more rational than segmental arterial stripping.[51] In 1991 an important series of studies on monkeys by Kaarela and colleagues[52] did not show complete loss of adrenergic innervation in the vasculature distal to the operative site after a 1-cm perivascular sympathectomy in the common volar vessels. Only the operative site itself and a few millimeters distally had complete loss of catecholamine fluorescence. Quantitative measurement of catecholamines in rabbit ear vessels after perivascular sympathectomy by the same investigators showed response to be lower in the distal segment when compared with the control side, but still about 9 times higher than at the sympathectomy site itself.[53]

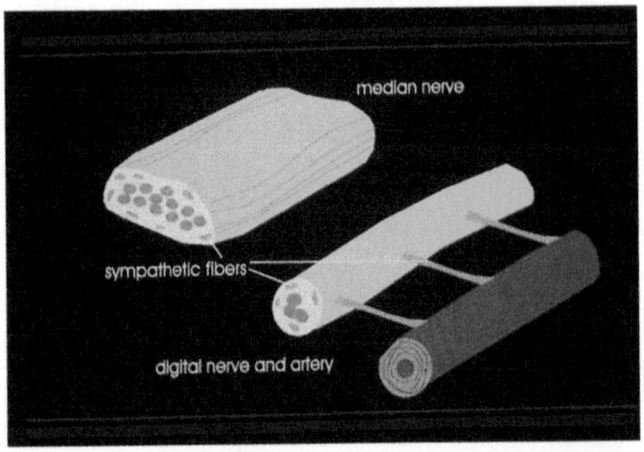

Fig. 6. Arterial muscle can only vasoconstrict in response to the segmental innervation from adjacent nerves.

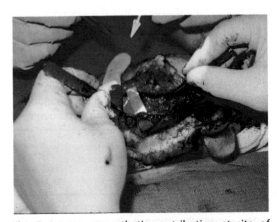

Fig. 7. Intense sympathetic contribution at site of bifurcation of the common volar artery into the proper digital artery.

Furthermore, comparison of the ulnar artery in scleroderma patients using color duplex ultrasonography shows significantly decreased blood flow velocity and significantly higher resistive indices than in controls.[54] It may therefore be concluded that periarterial sympathectomy (adventectomy) removes the sympathetic innervation at the site of surgery itself, and to a lesser extent reduces sympathetic activity distally, but would not be expected to alter any sympathetic response proximal to the site of surgery.

We therefore reason that a more extensive ("extended") perivascular sympathectomy of arteries that are likely to occlude may offer preventive measures at these sites, such as the ulnar artery in the distal forearm (including the nerve of Henle), the wrist, the proximal palm, and all of the common volar and proper digital vessels, in addition to the dorsal radial artery. Flatt[7] performed distal sympathectomy at the level of the bifurcation of the common into the proper digital arteries, stripping only a 3- to 4-mm segment of adventitia under $2\times$ magnification. We now reason that a much more extensive dissection is needed in patients with connective tissue disease to prevent later proximal occlusion. This fact seems especially relevant if the mechanism for endovascular thickening is reperfusion injury associated with chronic Raynaud attacks.

SURGICAL INDICATIONS

In our early experience, most patients with Raynaud syndrome were referred for amputations, with gangrenous changes often present for months. We knew that simple amputation would result in necrosis and failed healing of the amputation stump, leading to a more proximal amputation (see **Fig. 1**). This sequence has been reversed by adjunctive periarterial sympathectomies, and sometimes revascularization (when the ulnar or radial artery is occluded) at the time of initial debridement and amputation, permitting removal of only devitalized tissue, usually with predictable healing of the amputation stump (**Fig. 8**).

Because of doubts regarding any long-term value of periarterial sympathectomy for patients with connective tissue disease, our earlier indications for surgery required impending ischemic necrosis or gangrenous change. Over the years, observation of the profound and seemingly sustained surgical benefit has led us to change our criteria to include any patient who has unremitting ischemic pain that is not manageable by pharmacologic or hand therapy measures. It is preferable to operate before any ischemic necrosis occurs.

Wilgis[55] and others suggested combining digital plethysmography with cold stress testing using bupivacaine blocks at the palmar area as a criterion to determine the potential benefit of surgery. We have seen patients with ischemic necrosis who did not respond to blocks, but did benefit from digital sympathectomy, as have Zachary and colleagues,[56] Koman and colleagues[57] and Yee and colleagues,[58] so we consider that patients should not be excluded from surgery by this test. However, Botox injection may prove an excellent criterion for the response of sympathectomy. We have seen dramatic relief from ischemic discomfort, and have used Botox as a practical measure for amputations or elective digital surgery when an extended periarterial sympathectomy was not desired, permitting healing of the amputation stump without precipitating an ischemic attack. Botox injection may negate the need for sympathectomy in many patients, as suggested by Van Beek (Van Beek A, personal communication, 2006) and Neumeister (Neumeister M, personal communication, 2012), but it will not correct proximally occluded vessels, and these patients are less likely to respond.

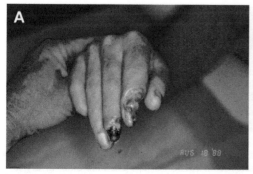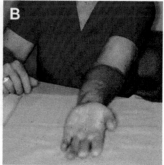

Fig. 8. A patient with mixed connective tissue disease (*A*) with occluded ulnar artery had primary healing of amputations following vein-graft reconstruction and extended periarterial sympathectomies (*B*).

PERIARTERIAL SYMPATHECTOMY: SURGICAL TECHNIQUES

Although there are relatively few reports on long-term benefits of digital artery sympathectomy, these describe longer-lasting benefits and less morbidity in comparison with reports on cervico-thoracic sympathectomy in patients with connective tissue disease[2,7,8,40,42,58–63]; however, there is little consensus on how the operation should be done in regard to which digits and the extent of dissection (see **Table 1**). Some surgeons confine the surgical approach to only the painfully ischemic or gangrenous digits,[40,55,60,61,64] stripping the distal common volar vessels and proper digital vessels to the level of the proximal inter-phalangeal joint. This approach is a good option for patients with injury to specific digits, such as frostbite or trauma, but affords no prophylactic benefit to avoid reoperation in patients with progressive connective tissue disease, such as scleroderma or lupus. Levine and colleagues,[65] Jones and colleagues,[66] Zachary and colleagues,[56] and others have used a more extensive procedure, including the other digits, while still confining their efforts to the common volar and proper vessels. El-Gammal and Blair[62] included adventectomy of a segment of the radial and ulnar vessels in addition to common volar and proper digital arteries using multiple vertical incisions, but omitting the superficial arch. Koman and colleagues[57] included 2-cm segments of the radial and ulnar vessels of the wrist and the dorsal radial artery in the snuffbox, as well as the superficial arch at the take-off of the common volar vessels. O'Brien and colleagues[42] described a more aggressive approach, stripping the ulnar artery at the wrist, superficial arch, and common volar and proper digital vessels well into the fingers of all of the digits. Some of these cases were done as a staged procedure.

Evolution of Extended Periarterial Sympathectomy and Technical Considerations

In our early digital artery sympathectomy experience in patients with connective tissue disease, reoperations led to the more aggressive approach we call extended periarterial sympathectomy. At the time of amputations in our early cases we stripped vessels to all 4 fingers using a transverse palmar incision, with a 2- to 3-cm segment involving the common volar vessels to their bifurcation into proper digital arteries, which in those days we thought was an aggressive amount of adventectomy. Our surgical criteria required either painful ischemic ulceration or frank gangrene. We were initially pleased, and presented our first 15 patients in 1985,[67] with no recurring ulcerations in operated hands and primary healing of amputation stumps. However, some of these patients later developed painful ischemic change in operated hands owing to ulnar artery occlusion at or proximal to the wrist (**Fig. 9**).

We then performed end-to-side vein-graft bypass reconstruction of the occluded ulnar artery to the superficial vascular arch distally before they developed new ulcerations or gangrene. Dissection of the superficial arch was tedious because of the previous surgery, so now we include the patent ulnar artery at initial operation, stripping its adventitia in the distal one-third of the forearm including the area supplied by the nerve of Henle,[46,47] in addition to the wrist, palm, and digital vessels. This prophylactic periarterial stripping of the ulnar artery seems to have protected our patients, with only one late occlusion following the procedure in a scleroderma patient who continued to smoke and use vibratory tools in a landscaping business, occluding his ulnar artery 4 years following sympathectomy. He had vein-graft reconstruction and abandoned the landscaping business.

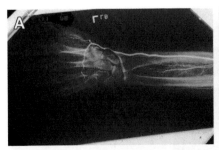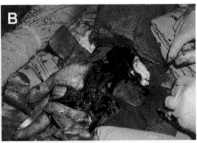

Fig. 9. (*A*) Ulnar artery occlusion years after palmar periarterial sympathectomy in scleroderma patient. (*B*) Surgical repair with a 15-cm end-to-side vein-graft reconstruction of the occluded ulnar artery to the superficial arch. ([*B*] *From* Merritt WH, Masear VR. Reoperative hand surgery. In: Grotting JC, editor. Reoperative aesthetic & reconstructive plastic surgery. St Louis (MO): QMP; 2007. p. 1902; with permission.)

Subsequently, we encountered patients with connective tissue disease who developed late postoperative problems in their index and thumb digits, which responded to periarterial dorsal radial artery sympathectomy from the level of the snuffbox distally to where the vessels bifurcate and go beneath the first dorsal interosseous muscle to form the deep palmar arch. One early patient developed radial artery occlusion after sympathectomy that had not included the radial artery, and 2 presented initially with occlusions that required vein-graft reconstructions (**Fig. 10**).

Therefore, we now also include the dorsal radial artery in the initial stripping. These experiences led to our current philosophy in patients with connective tissue disease, which is in keeping with the studies of Kaarela and colleagues[52] in monkeys, showing protection from vasoconstriction only at the level of surgery and to a limited extent distally, but no protection from proximal vasoconstriction. Given that postmortem studies in scleroderma patients suggest almost half may develop occlusion of the ulnar artery,[19,42,64,68] primary periarterial sympathectomy of this vessel in the forearm and wrist may avoid a more difficult and tedious procedure in the future. Although radial artery occlusion is less frequent, adventectomy is easier than reconstruction, so our primary operation now includes both ulnar and dorsal radial arteries in patients with connective tissue disease.

Current Recommended Technique

In patients with connective tissue disease our primary operation now includes adventectomy of the dorsal branch of the radial artery from the snuffbox to its passage into branches beneath the first dorsal interosseous, the ulnar artery from a point approximately 8 to 10 cm proximal to the wrist crease, up to and including the entire superficial vascular arch, the common volar vessels preserving the communicating branches from the deep

vascular arch (sometimes at their bifurcation), and the proper digital arteries to all fingers about 3 to 5 mm distal from the common volar bifurcation into the base of the digit (**Fig. 11**). When ischemic necrosis or gangrene is present, we now usually include the proper digital arteries in the afflicted digit to the level of the proximal interphalangeal joint if they are patent (**Fig. 12**). We consider that high-risk vessels may be protected from occlusion by early adventectomy, and the results of this extended, more aggressive approach have been rewarding.

Anesthesia and Incisions

General or axillary block anesthesia is used, and the potential value of the periarterial sympathectomy becomes evident as soon as the patient is induced or blocked, because digits that previously were cyanotic become pink in the operating room. Doppler reassessment is more convenient at this time than before anesthesia for a more accurate appraisal. We now prefer 2 incisions because of some early problems with an L-shaped flap that developed necrosis at its tip (none of which required secondary surgery). One is a distal transverse incision 1 to 1.5 cm proximal to the finger flexion creases, and the second a vertical incision made in the central palm placed with approximately a 1-cm bridge of skin between the 2 incisions and exposing the entire vasculature (**Fig. 13**). The vertical incision originates in the central palm, then borders the hypothenar eminence in line with the level used for carpal tunnel release. At the wrist crease it is angled ulnarly and thereafter vertically along the ulnar artery in the forearm for approximately 8 to 10 cm in routine cases. Intraoperative Doppler mapping of the ulnar artery is of assistance in placing this incision.

The initial incisions, flap elevation, and isolation of the neurovascular bundles using small vascular loops are made under tourniquet control and

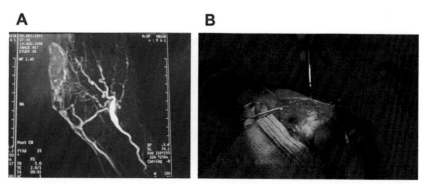

Fig. 10. (*A*) Dorsal radial artery occlusion 12 years after ulnar artery vein graft, which is still patent. (*B*) Radial artery vein-graft reconstruction used to relieve thumb and index vasospasm.

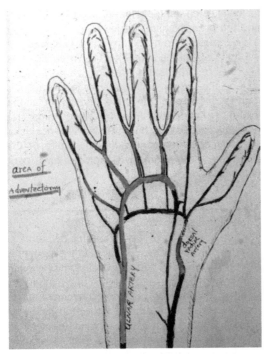

Fig. 11. Extended periarterial sympathectomy (*green area*) includes distal one-third of the ulnar artery in the forearm and the entire superficial arch, common volar vessels, and proper digital arteries into the digits and the dorsal radial artery.

4× loupe magnification; the remaining dissection and vascular reconstruction is done without tourniquet using the microscope because it is easier to determine the amount of adventitia that can be safely stripped from diseased vessels during blood flow. Ophthalmic Vannas scissors are useful to strip, push, and pull the adventitia circumferentially away from the vessel (**Fig. 14**, Video 1), and an ophthalmic muscle hook helps retract vessels as they are stripped circumferentially. The greatest concentration of sympathetic neurofilaments will be found at the bifurcations in the superficial vascular arch (Video 2) and at the termination of

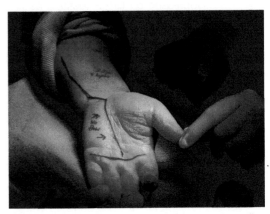

Fig. 13. Two preferred incisions to prevent flap necrosis.

the common volar vessels (Video 3), and at the wrist and distal forearm levels. Additional time spent at these sites is worthwhile.

The dorsal radial artery is exposed with incision on the dorsum of the thumb web, extending to the snuffbox, and adventitia is stripped from the level of the snuffbox, beneath the extensor pollicis longus, and as far distally as possible until the vessels branch and become inaccessible beneath the first dorsal interosseous muscle. We encountered 3 patients with occluded radial arteries who had vein-graft reconstruction, and found that they reconstituted from collaterals at the distal level, where careful dissection allows distal arterial elevation at the site of branching to perform a difficult end-to-side anastomosis. The vein grafts were placed over the extensor pollicis longus tendon to avoid any possibility of future compression beneath it (see **Fig. 10**B).

VEIN-GRAFT RECONSTRUCTIONS ASSOCIATED WITH PERIARTERIAL SYMPATHECTOMY

Because of the high incidence of ulnar artery occlusion (50%) in scleroderma patients,

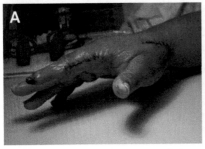
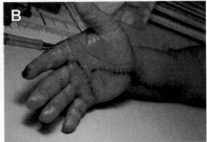

Fig. 12. (*A*, *B*) Periarterial sympathectomy extended to proximal interphalangeal joint level in digits with ischemic necrosis.

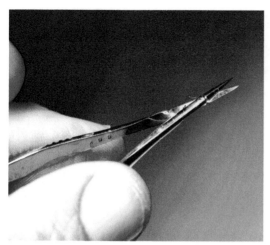

Fig. 14. Vannas scissors are useful for adventitial stripping because of the triangular shape of the blade (see Video 1).

reconstruction of this vessel is a frequent technical consideration. Approximately 20% of our patients are referred with their ulnar artery already occluded, and reverse vein-graft reconstruction is indicated, along with extended periarterial sympathectomy. Jones and colleagues[68] and Koman and colleagues[57] described replacing the entire superficial vascular arch by end-to-end vein graft to the proximal ulnar artery with common volar vessels microvascularly reinserted into the vein graft (often the saphenous). In Jones'[69] series of 14 patients with occlusion from various causes, recurrent ulceration occurred in 20%, with occlusion of the graft in 35%.

In most of our patients with ulnar occlusion, collateral circulation to the superficial vascular arch was audible because of communicating branches from the deep to the superficial arch, although this was not always visualized on radiographic study.[70] We have been able to use an end-to-side method for vein-graft reconstruction of occluded ulnar vessels in most patients, thereby preserving the collateral circulation with what appears to be reduced incidence of recurrent ulceration and occlusion than that reported elsewhere (**Fig. 15**). We are not aware of any patient losing a digit in approximately 30 cases of vascular reconstruction, but a few occluded the vein graft without any apparent adverse effect. One patient with associated cryoglobulinemia had reoperative surgery for symptomatic vein-graft occlusion. We now maintain vein-grafted patients on clopidogrel and have documented long-term patency. In fact, one lupus patient with 4 vein grafts has remained patent for 16 years (**Fig. 16**). Savvidou and Tsai[71] agreed with the value of periarterial sympathectomy at the time of vascular reconstruction, even in patients who do not have connective tissue disease.

At the time of vein grafting it is useful to distend the venous segment to be grafted with heparinized saline, and dot the surface with methylene blue before harvesting to avoid twisting the graft. Mostly the cephalic vein is used, with the median antecubital vein or the basilic vein used less frequently. Vein-graft branches are suture ligated on the side of the vessel using interrupted 9-0 nylon sutures, and vascular clips are used on the distal portion of these branches. A curved vascular clamp is placed on the distal end and a straight clamp on the proximal end to remind us to reverse the graft in its new position. All our vein grafts have been harvested from the volar forearm, commonly the cephalic vessel, and have varied from 6 to 15 cm in length. We never use the saphenous vein, but one scleroderma patient with severe skin induration had her ulnar artery vena comitans utilized for grafting.

We now also include a regimen of dripping Botox solution on the vein graft and the exposed arterial vasculature because of our impression that the vein graft has less traumatic vasospasm after this

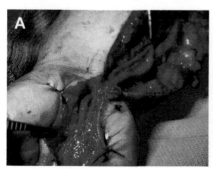
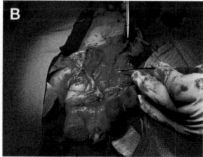

Fig. 15. (*A*) Proximal ulnar artery vein graft anastomosis (ulnar artery vein-graft reconstruction using "Hunnius" Rummel-type vascular control, with clamps out of the microscopic field). (*B*) Distal vein graft anastomosis to superficial arch.

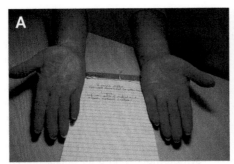
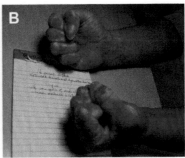

Fig. 16. (*A, B*) Sixteen years after bilateral dorsal radial artery and ulnar artery vein grafts in a lupus patient who had ischemic necrosis (anticoagulated).

maneuver, and our laboratory studies show long-term arterial response.[72] The arterial incision for vein-graft reconstruction is done with a small pointed Alcon Beaver blade (**Fig. 17**) and the end-to-side anastomosis performed with 10-0 nylon at the distal end of the reverse vein graft. This anastomosis being the more difficult one, it is done first. Many times the superficial arch lumen is narrowed from the thickened wall, and a 1.00-mm Flo-Rester vessel occluder is often useful when placing the initial distal end-to-side sutures to protect patency (see **Fig. 17**). Doppler assessment will assist in determining the best site for anastomosis along the superficial arterial arch.

We developed a Rummel-type impecunious (cheap) vascular occlusion system that has proved to be safe and easy to use, which we affectionately call the "Hunnius clamp" after the nurse who scavenged the simple, inexpensive components. This procedure is done using microvascular right-angle forceps to loop Sterion silicone microvessel tubing around the vessels to be controlled, and

placing a segment of #8 Red Robinson pediatric catheter over the ends of the microvessel loops by means of a #7 tonsil snare wire (**Fig. 18**). Once the loops are through the tubing, a Hartman mosquito clamp can be used to cinch this down to occlude the vessel (**Fig. 19**). Sufficient catheter length can be used to place the clamp outside the microsurgical field, facilitating the anastomosis; this is particularly valuable when there is an anastomotic leak that obscures vessels needing to be reclamped. Small collateral branches beneath the vessel to be sutured are more easily occluded with small microvascular clamps positioned so that they do not interfere with the anastomosis.

The proximal anastomosis is usually sutured with interrupted 9-0 microvascular sutures after resecting a small ellipse of arterial wall using angled Vannas scissors. The vein graft is beveled,

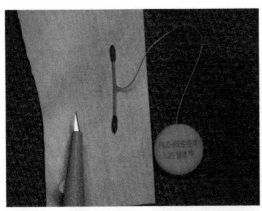

Fig. 17. Flo-Rester to assist distal anastomosis, and a knife for distal arteriotomy. (*Courtesy of* Synovis Surgical Innovations, Synovis Life Technologies, St Paul, MN; with permission.)

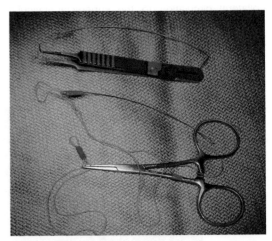

Fig. 18. Right-angle microvascular forceps, Sterion silicone microvessel tubing threaded through #8 red Robinson pediatric catheter segment, and Hartman mosquito forceps to create Rummel-type vascular control.

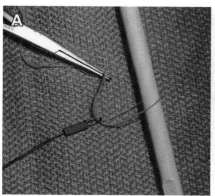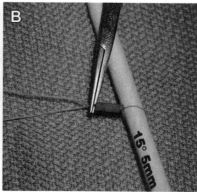

Fig. 19. The #7 tonsil snare wire is used to thread the silicone tubing through the segment of pediatric catheter (*A*), then cinched down onto the vessel with the Hartman forceps (*B*).

and both distal and proximal anastomoses are completed before release of the Rummel-type Hunnius clamps. It is preferable to place the vein graft on slight tension at the proximal anastomosis, because even though it may seem to be under tension, it will lengthen as soon as blood flow is restored. Patency is confirmed with a Hayhurst test, although pulsatile blood flow through the vein graft is usually apparent.

Even though a large segment of occluded ulnar artery may be bypassed by the vein graft, we consider it important to strip adventitia from the occluded portion of the vessel along with the other vessels sympathectomized. We reason that early surgery for hypothenar hammer syndrome was simply by excising the occluded segment of ulnar artery, which gave relief from ischemia and Raynaud phenomenon. Although this prevented further emboli, it is also possible that sympathetic stimulation from the occluded vessel played a role, and we suspect that resection of the occluded segment may give relief by means of sympathectomy.[57] Although the value of this additional adventectomy is uncertain, it seems prudent and is easier than resection of the occluded segment. This extended technique for periarterial sympathectomy is reserved for patients thought to have scleroderma or other connective tissue disease, and its greatest advantage may prove to be its early use to reduce or prevent further predictable occlusion.

Closure is done using 3-0 chromic sutures for the dermal layer in the forearm and dorsum of the hand, and interrupted 4-0 Prolene for skin incisions. Marcaine is injected along the median and ulnar nerves first at the wrist level, then in the superficial radial nerve on the hand to reduce postoperative discomfort. Drains are not usually necessary, but are used if there is undue oozing in the palm. The hand is immobilized in a soft dressing with tongue-blade splint, maintaining the wrist in approximately 15° to 20° of extension, with the metacarpophalangeal joints flexed and the interphalangeal joints extended.

Patients are given ketorolac before the end of the procedure to reduce postoperative discomfort and to discourage platelet aggregation. Patients with vein grafts are maintained on clopidogrel postoperatively, and those who have not had vein grafts are on aspirin. The patients are usually outpatients, unless a vascular reconstruction is done (approximately one-fifth), in which case they are observed overnight.

POSTOPERATIVE MANAGEMENT

Following surgery, the patient is at rest with the hand elevated until the fourth or fifth day, when hand therapy is instituted. Stiffness is common, but therapy sometimes recovers better motion than preoperatively. In general, however, the goal is to recover the preoperative range of motion. When sensation was diminished preoperatively, we generally measure improvement following surgery. The therapist uses a resting splint and encourages active motion recovery with use of the hand to the extent that it is comfortable. Most recover motion quickly, but those with sclerodactyly will have greater stiffness and a longer therapy regimen. Patients with a vein graft are not allowed out of their protective wrist splint until after the 10th postoperative day.

Not infrequently, temporary neurapraxia occurs, and patients are reassured and monitored until they have recovered full sensation. It is surprising how little these patients complain of postoperative pain. Therapy is continued until after patients have recovered full amplitude of motion and full sensation, which varies from 3 weeks to as much as

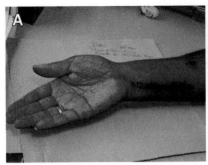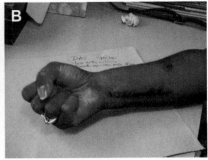

Fig. 20. (*A, B*) Scleroderma patient 18 years after surgery following extended periarterial sympathectomy and ulnar artery vein grafting with hypertrophic scarring.

12 weeks, especially in sclerodactyly patients with postoperative stiffness.

OUTCOMES

All patients seem to experience relief from severe ischemic pain, usually immediately after surgery. Although there were no intraoperative or perioperative deaths, more than 20% of these patients have died during the late follow-up interval (up to 33 years), which likely represents the seriousness of the disease process. Although patients report subjective relief and have improved sensory measurements and enhanced nail growth, most continue to remain cold sensitive and still vulnerable to Raynaud attacks, reportedly less frequently and less severe. A few report complete relief. Some formed hypertrophic scars but still had a favorable long-term result (**Fig. 20**). Several have had transient episodes of paronychia, sometimes stubborn, which respond to conservative management using topical gentian violet dye. Our dialysis patients with ischemia have not done as well as the patients with connective tissue disease.

LONG-TERM RESULTS

Several years ago Jonathan Isaacs surveyed a group of our patients during his orthopedic surgery training more than a decade ago, studying 21 patients after 31 sympathectomies.[73] The long-term results were better than expected. Average follow-up was 7 years, with follow-up of up to 14 years, and the average age at surgery was 27 years (18–87 years), with twice as many women as men. A favorable follow-up was reported for 28 of the 31 operated hands, with 2 of the unfavorable results in the same scleroderma patient, a persistent heavy cigarette smoker. Both patients with failures had sufficient severity that amputations were necessary at initial surgery.

When he studied recurrent ulceration, 77% of the patients remained improved or asymptomatic, and 83% of those who were surveyed more than 5 years after surgery had remained improved or asymptomatic. In answer to questions about ischemic pain, 90% of the patients stated they were improved or asymptomatic compared with the preoperative status, and this was true in 86% who were surveyed more than 5 years after surgery.

It is possible that patients with more serious disease involvement may have died, so that the long-term results represent patients with a more favorable course, but these surprising long-term beneficial results have encouraged the concept of earlier extensive periarterial sympathectomy to reduce the pattern of vasospasm and reperfusion injury, creating less frequent and less severe Raynaud attacks. The findings suggest a surprising degree of benefit longer than 5 years after surgery in patients with previous medical failure.

Without controls, it is difficult to prove that the extended periarterial sympathectomy altered the outcome in these patients, but if one reviews the history of Raynaud syndrome in patients with connective tissue disease under medical management, the incidence of ischemic ulceration is reported to be as high as 20% to 30% per year,[74] and ulnar artery occlusion is common, as high as 50% in scleroderma patients.[19,42,68] Given that this surgical series selected unfavorable patients with advanced disease who had already become medical failures, their 86% postoperative relief of ischemic pain and 83% decreased incidence of recurrent ulceration or gangrene more than 5 years after surgery has enhanced our support and belief in this procedure as more than palliation.

SUMMARY

It should be pointed out that extended periarterial sympathectomy is for patients with either known or suspected connective tissue disease, and not for patients with hypothenar hammer syndrome, emboli, aneurysm, frostbite, or other causes of Raynaud syndrome. Although the pattern of vasospastic attacks may be similar, patients with hypothenar hammer syndrome need only the offending segment of vessel resected and replaced. Many of the symptoms from hypothenar hammer syndrome, radial artery occlusion, or aneurysms may derive from emboli, so it is important to resect the damaged segment of vasculature (**Fig. 21**). Patients with the gradual occlusion associated with Raynaud syndrome in connective tissue disease have vessel-wall thickening and narrowed lumens, but do not seem to experience emboli.

Patients with Raynaud syndrome from cryoglobulinemia associated with malignancy may have multiple areas of microvascular occlusion, but even these patients seem to improve from perivascular sympathectomy and topical Botox application. In one patient with occult myeloma causing unrecognized cryoglobulinemia, 2 ulnar artery vein grafts and 1 radial artery vein graft were done after initial periarterial sympathectomy for recurrent symptoms over a 12-year interval until the diagnosis was finally made by bone marrow biopsy (there were no manifestations other than cryoglobulinemia), and the patient remained pain-free without further difficulty on anticoagulation. Patients with Raynaud syndrome following digital trauma need only the involved digits treated by periarterial sympathectomy; a Botox injection trial may afford some prognostication about possible surgical benefit, and may actually be all that is needed for some patients. Our few patients with

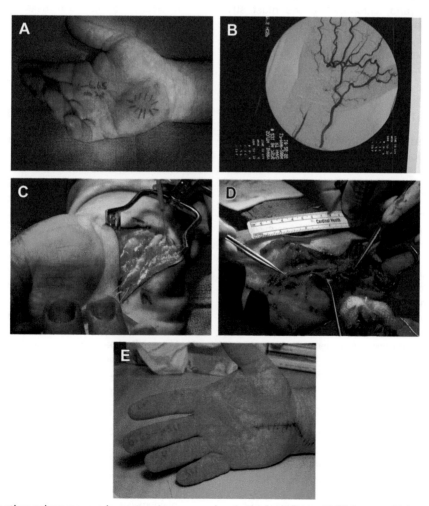

Fig. 21. Hypothenar hammer syndrome causing sensory loss in the long finger (6.65 Semmes-Weinstein monofilament measurements) (*A*), evident on arteriography (*B*). (*C, D*) Occluded segment resected and replaced with reverse cephalic end-to-end vein graft. (*E*) Sensory recovery in early postoperative interval (3.61 Semmes-Weinstein monofilament measurements).

Buerger disease seem to benefit from extended periarterial sympathectomy, at least initially, but long-term results will likely vary according to nicotine use. Those without significant gangrene have rewarding nonsurgical treatment with only Botox injection and nicotine abstinence.

Although most clinicians still regard surgery for Raynaud syndrome as a salvage procedure[57] in patients who do not respond to pharmacologic or physical medicine management, experience with newer microvascular surgical techniques on distal vessels seems to offer improved benefit and less morbidity than previous proximal sympathectomy procedures, and our long-term follow-up suggests that later vasospastic occlusion may be reduced or prevented in patients with connective tissue disease. However, the appropriate role, timing, indications, and techniques for perivascular distal sympathectomy are still evolving, and, unfortunately, we must still agree with Maurice Raynaud's original observation in 1862: "I hope that it will be readily understood that for a disease, so many aspects of which are still obscure, I cannot formulate a complete treatment."

SUPPLEMENTARY DATA

Videos related to this article can be found online at http://dx.doi.org/10.1016/j.hcl.2014.09.011.

REFERENCES

1. Raynaud M. De l'Asphyxie locale et de la gangrene symetrique des extremities. [On local asphyxia and symmetrical gangrene of the extremities]. Paris: Leclerc; Rignoux, publ; 1862.
2. Belch JF, Sturrock RD. Raynaud's syndrome: current trends. Br J Rheumatol 1983;22:50–5.
3. Coffman JD. Raynaud's phenomenon: an update. Hypertension 1991;17:593–602.
4. Roath S. Management of Raynaud's phenomenon: focus on newer treatments. Drugs 1989;37:700–12.
5. Wollersheim I, Cleophas T, Thien T. The role of a sympathetic nervous system in the pathophysiology and therapy of Raynaud's phenomenon. Vasa Suppl 1987;18:54–63.
6. Skotnicki S, VanDeWal H, Lacqet L, et al. Treatment of patients with Raynaud's phenomenon by thoracic sympathectomy. Vasa Suppl 1987;18:42–7.
7. Flatt A. Digital artery sympathectomy. J Hand Surg Am 1980;5:550–6.
8. Merritt WH. Comprehensive management of Raynaud's syndrome. Clin Plast Surg 1997;24(1):146.
9. Lewis T. Experiments relating to the peripheral mechanism involved in spasmodic arrest of the circulation in the finger: a variety of Raynaud's disease. Heart 1929;15:7–101.
10. Friedman RR, Ianni P. Role of cold and emotional stress in Raynaud's disease and scleroderma. Br Med J (Clin Res Ed) 1983;287:1499–502.
11. Fagius J, Blumberg H. Sympathetic outflow in the hand in patients with Raynaud's phenomenon. Cardiovasc Res 1985;19:249.
12. Sapira JD, Rodnan GP, Scheib ET, et al. Studies of endogenous catecholamines in patients with Raynaud's phenomenon secondary to progressive systemic sclerosis (scleroderma). Am J Med 1972;52:330–7.
13. Kahaleh B, Matucci-Cerinic M. Raynaud's phenomenon in scleroderma: dysregulated neuroendothelial control of vascular control. Arthritis Rheum 1995;38:1–4.
14. Levine JD, Goetzl EJ, Vasbaum AI. Contribution of the nervous system to the pathophysiology of rheumatoid arthritis and other polyarthritides. Rheum Dis Clin North Am 1987;13:369.
15. Wallengren J, Ekman R, Sundler F. Occurrence and distribution of neuropeptides in human skin: an immunocytochemical and immunochemical study of normal skin and blister fluid from inflamed skin. Acta Derm Venereol 1987;67:185–92.
16. Bunker CB, Reavley C, O'Shaughnessy DJ, et al. Calcitonin gene-related peptide in treatment of severe peripheral insufficiency in Raynaud's phenomenon. Lancet 1993;342:80–3.
17. Priollet T, Vayssairat M, Housset E. How to classify Raynaud's phenomenon. Am J Med 1987;83:491–8.
18. Blunt RJ, Porter JM. Raynaud's syndrome. Semin Arthritis Rheum 1981;10:282–308.
19. Rodman GP, Myerowitz RL, Jusch GO. Morphological changes in the digital arteries of patients with progressive systemic sclerosis (scleroderma) and Raynaud's phenomenon. Medicine 1980;59:393.
20. Marcus S, Weiner SR, Suzuki SM, et al. Raynaud's syndrome: using a range of therapies to help patients. Postgrad Med 1991;89:171–87.
21. Miller NE. Learning of visceral and glandular responses. Science 1969;163:434–45.
22. Jobe JB, Sampson JB, Roberts DE, et al. Induced vasodilatation as a treatment for Raynaud's disease. Ann Intern Med 1982;97:706–9.
23. McIntyre DR. A manoeuvre to reverse Raynaud's phenomenon of the fingers. JAMA 1978;240:2760.
24. Zhong J. Clinical applications of accupoint. J Tradit Chin Med 1993;13:205–6.
25. Kaada B. Vasodilatation induced by transcutaneous nerve stimulation in peripheral ischemia (Raynaud's phenomenon and diabetic polyneuropathy). Eur Heart J 1982;3:303–14.
26. Bonica JJ, Buckley FP. Regional anesthesia with local anesthetics. In: Bonica JJ, editor. The

management of pain. Malvern (PA): Lea & Febiger; 1990. p. 1935–6.

27. Francaviglia N, Sylvestro C, Maiello M, et al. Spinal cord stimulation for the treatment of progressive systemic sclerosis and Raynaud's syndrome. Br J Neurosurg 1994;8:567–73.

28. Kiowski W, Erne P, Buhler FR. Use of nifedipine in hypertension and Raynaud's phenomenon. Cardiovasc Drugs Ther 1990;4(Suppl 5):935–40.

29. Coffman JD. New drug therapy in peripheral vascular disease. Med Clin North Am 1988;72:259–65.

30. Moriau M, Lavenne-Pardonge E, Crasborn L, et al. Treatment of Raynaud's phenomenon with piracetam. Arzneimittelforschung 1993;43:526–35.

31. Seibold JR. Serotonin in Raynaud's phenomenon. J Cardiovasc Pharmacol 1985;7(Suppl):95–8.

32. Sycha T, Graninger M, Auff E, et al. Botulinum toxin in the treatment of Raynaud's phenomenon: a pilot study. Eur J Clin Invest 2004;34(4):312–3.

33. Stadlmaier E, Müller T, Hermann J, et al. Raynaud's phenomenon: treatment with botulinum toxin. Ann Rheum Dis 2005;64(Suppl III):275.

34. Neumeister M, Gillespie J, Chambers C. Botox therapy for ischemic digits. Can J Plast Surg 2006;14(2):97.

35. Bank J, Fuller S, Henry G, et al. Fat grafting to the hand in patients with Raynaud phenomenon: a novel therapeutic modality. Plast Reconstr Surg 2014;133(5):1109–18.

36. Sultan SM, Stern CS, Allen RJ Jr, et al. Human fat grafting alleviates radiation skin damage in a murine model. Plast Reconstr Surg 2011;128:363–72.

37. Maricq HR, Weinrich MC. Diagnostic aids called 100% sensitive, specific for Raynaud's. Skin/Allergy News 1988;19:28.

38. Porter J, Snyder R, Bardana E, et al. The diagnosis and treatment of Raynaud's phenomenon. Surgery 1975;771:11–23.

39. Delp HI, Newton RA. Effects of brief cold exposure on finger dexterity and sensibility in subjects with Raynaud's phenomenon. Phys Ther 1986;66:503–7.

40. Miller LM, Morgan RF. Vasospastic disorders. Hand Clin 1993;9:171–87.

41. Kransdorf MJ, Turner-Stepahin S, Merritt W. MR angiography of the hand and wrist, value in the evaluation of patients with severe ischemic disease. J Reconstr Microsurg 1998;14(2):77–81.

42. O'Brien BM, Kumar PA, Mellow CG, et al. Radical microarteriolysis in the treatment of vasospastic disorders of the hand, especially scleroderma. J Hand Surg Br 1992;17:447–52.

43. McGrath MA, Penny R. The mechanism of Raynaud's phenomenon: part II. Med J Aust 1974;2:367–75.

44. Arnulf G. Physiological basis of sympathetic surgery for the upper limb in Raynaud's diseases. J Cardiovasc Surg 1976;17:354–7.

45. Pick J. The autonomic nervous system. Philadelphia: JB Lippincott; 1970.

46. Balogh B, Valencak J, Vesely M, et al. The nerve of Henle: an anatomic and immunohistochemical study. J Hand Surg Am 1999;24(5):1103–8.

47. McCabe SJ, Kleinert JM. The nerve of Henle. J Hand Surg Am 1990;15(5):784–8.

48. Mitchell G. Anatomy of the autonomic nervous system. Edinburgh (Scotland): ES Livingston; 1953.

49. Morgan R, Reisman N, Wilgis F. Anatomic localization of sympathetic nerves in the hand. J Hand Surg Am 1983;8:283–8.

50. Morgan R, Wilgis F. Thermal changes in a rabbit car model after sympathectomy. J Hand Surg Am 1986;11:120–6.

51. Miller G, Kaufman M. Periarterial sympathectomy. Can Med Assoc J 1928;18(4):425–7.

52. Kaarela O, Raatikainen T, Carlson S, et al. Effect of perivascular sympathectomy on distal adrenergic innervation in the hand of monkeys. J Hand Surg Br 1991;16:386–8.

53. Kaarela O, Huttunen P, Junita J, et al. The effects of perivascular sympathectomy to the noradrenaline content of the distal vasculature in rabbit ears. Eur J Plast Surg 1991;14(6):285–7.

54. Frerix M, Steghauer J, Dragun D, et al. Ulnar artery occlusion is predictive of digital ulcers in SSc. Rheumatology 2012;51(4):735–42.

55. Wilgis ES. Evaluation and Treatment of chronic digital ischemia. Ann Surg 1981;193:693–8.

56. Zachary LS, Tinsley ZX, Ellman M. Microscopic digital sympathectomy in scleroderma. Presented at ASSH. San Francisco, CA, September 1995.

57. Koman A, Ruch D, Smith VP, et al. Vascular disorders. In: David Green, editor. Green's operative hand surgery. vol. 2. Edinburgh (Scotland): Churchill-Livingstone; 1999. p. 2296.

58. Yee AM, Hotchkiss RN, Paget SA. Adventitial stripping: a digit-saving procedure in refractory Raynaud's phenomenon. J Rheumatol 1998;25(2):269–76.

59. Birnstingl M. Results of sympathectomy in digital artery disease. BMJ 1967;2:601.

60. Drake D, Morgan R. Digital sympathectomy for refractory Raynaud's in an adolescent. J Rheumatol 1992;19:1286–8.

61. Egloff DV, Mifsud RP, Verdan CL. Superselective digital sympathectomy in Raynaud's phenomenon. Hand 1982;15:110–4.

62. El-Gammal TA, Blair WF. Digital periarterial sympathectomy for ischemic digital pain and ulcers. J Hand Surg Br 1991;16:382–5.

63. Balogh B, Mayer W, Vesely M, et al. Adventitial stripping of the radial and ulnar arteries in Raynaud's disease. J Hand Surg Am 2002;27(6):1073–80.

64. Hartzell T, Makhni E, Sampson C. Long-term results of periarterial sympathectomy. J Hand Surg Am 2009;34(8):1454–60.

65. Levine NS, Buchanan RT, Sanchez A, et al. Evaluation of an extended digital sympathectomy for vasospastic and vasoocclusive disease in the upper extremity. Presented at 14th annual meeting AAHS. Acapulco Princess Hotel, Acapulco, Mexico, November 25–29, 1984.

66. Jones NF, Imbrigha JE, Steen VD, et al. Surgery for scleroderma of the hand. J Hand Surg Am 1987; 12:391–400.

67. Carrico T, Merritt W. Digital artery for Raynaud's syndrome in connective tissue disease patients. Presented 1st annual meeting ASRM. Las Vegas, NV, September 1985.

68. Jones NF, Raynor SC, Medsger TA. Microsurgical revascularization of the hand in scleroderma. Br J Plast Surg 1987;40:264–9.

69. Jones N. Acute and chronic ischemia of the hand: pathophysiology, treatment and prognosis. J Hand Surg Am 1991;16:1074–83.

70. Yu HL, Chase RA, Strauch B. Vascular systems. In: Chase RA, editor. Atlas of hand anatomy and clinical implications. St Louis (MO): Mosby; 2004. p. 419.

71. Savvidou C, Tsai T. Long-term results of arterial sympathectomy and artery reconstruction with vein bypass technique as a salvage procedure for severe digital ischemia. Ann Plast Surg 2013; 70:168–71.

72. Arnold P, Merritt W, Rodeheaver GT, et al. Effects of perivascular botulinum toxin-A application on vascular smooth muscle and flap viability in the rat. Ann Plast Surg 2009;62(5):463–7.

73. Isaacs J. Presented at the annual meeting of the World Society of Reconstructive Microsurgery. Heidelberg, Germany, June 2003.

74. Seibold JR, Allegar NE. The treatment of Raynaud's phenomenon. Clin Dermatol 1994;12:312–21.

75. Morgan RF, Drake DB, Kesler RW. Digital sympathectomy for refractory Raynaud's phenomenon in an adolescent. J Rheum 1992;19(8): 1286–8.

76. From Merritt WH, Masear VR. Reoperative hand surgery. In: Grotting JC, editor. Reoperative aesthetic & reconstructive plastic surgery. St Louis (MO): QMP; 2007. p. 1863–927.

New Developments in Management of Vascular Pathology of the Upper Extremity

 CrossMark

Victor W. Wong, MD, Ryan D. Katz, MD,
James P. Higgins, MD*

KEYWORDS

- Angiography • Arteriography • Hypothenar hammer • Ischemia • Thrombosis • Vascular disease

KEY POINTS

- Understanding the utility and interpretation of upper extremity angiography is critical for hand surgeons treating vasoocclusive diseases of the hand.
- Angiography remains the gold standard for detailed imaging of the vascular system of the upper extremity.
- Vascular collateralization helps maintain perfusion to the hand and facilitates reconstruction of the upper extremity.
- Hand surgeons should view real-time sequential images if possible to gain the most information about timing and quality of vascular flow to the hand.
- Angiographic findings do not always correlate with clinical presentation and may overestimate the extent of disease.

INTRODUCTION

Vascular diseases of the upper extremities are uncommon but can cause significant morbidity and decreased quality of life.[1] Ischemic complications develop when blood supply fails to meet physiologic demand. Broadly, 3 major pathologic mechanisms may be involved: occlusive disease (eg, embolic and thrombotic), vasospastic disease (eg, Raynaud disease/phenomenon), or low-flow states (eg, cardiac failure and vasopressors). A combination of these factors is often responsible for a spectrum of clinical findings, ranging from cold intolerance to tissue loss. The treatment of vascular disorders of the upper extremity is often considered the sole purview of the hand surgery specialist. This responsibility requires familiarity with both the pathophysiology of vascular disease and appreciation of the utility and interpretation of common diagnostic tests.

Noninvasive imaging modalities play an important role in the diagnosis of upper extremity vascular disease.[2] These studies include surface Doppler evaluation, laser Doppler fluxmetry and perfusion imaging, segmental arterial pressures, digital plethysmography, ultrasound, and 3-phase radionuclide bone scanning.[2] CT angiography also provides a rapid, noninvasive option for vascular imaging of the upper extremity, particularly useful in the setting of trauma.[3,4] Recent advances in magnetic resonance angiography have improved its ability to provide dynamic high-

The authors have nothing to disclose.
Curtis National Hand Center, MedStar Union Memorial Hospital, 3333 North Calvert Street #200, Baltimore, MD 21218, USA
* Corresponding author.
E-mail address: anne.mattson@medstar.net

Hand Clin 31 (2015) 121–134
http://dx.doi.org/10.1016/j.hcl.2014.09.009
0749-0712/15/$ – see front matter © 2015 Elsevier Inc. All rights reserved.

hand.theclinics.com

resolution images without the need for ionizing radiation.[5] Although noninvasive studies provide low-morbidity alternatives for large-vessel imaging, angiography provides superior small-vessel (ie, palmar arch and common and proper digital arteries) visualization. It is for this reason that contrast arteriography remains the gold standard for diagnosing vascular disease.

Clinical arteriography was first developed in the 1920s by Moniz and dos Santos, who studied the cerebral circulation and aorta, respectively.[6] Over the next several decades, improvements in catheter-based imaging culminated with the 1956 Nobel Prize in Medicine awarded to Forssmann, Cournand, and Richards for their seminal work in cardiac catheterization. In the 1950s, Seldinger introduced percutaneous guide wire techniques, which further accelerated the development of angiography. In the 1960s, Dotter introduced the use of intravascular catheters and stents, and by the 1980s, interventional radiology was recognized as both a diagnostic and therapeutic tool.[7,8]

Current techniques for upper extremity arteriography often use the transfemoral, axillary, or brachial artery approaches.[9] A complete upper extremity examination requires examination from the thoracic aortic arch to the digital arteries. Although angiography may miss extraluminal disease, more subtle findings, such as extensive collateralization and retrograde filling, may indicate pathology that is better appreciated on time-lapse imaging. Angiographic results may be influenced by ambient temperature (affecting blood flow) and the use of vasodilators (eg, tolazoline, phentolamine, nitroglycerin, and papaverine) to decrease arterial spasm. The introduction of digital subtraction techniques (ie, removal or subtraction of precontrast nonvessel structures from the contrast injection image) has permitted the use of more dilute and reduced volumes of contrast agents.[10]

The remainder of this article focuses on both normal and pathologic vascular anatomy from the aortic arch to the digital vessels and presents practical tips for maximizing the utility of diagnostic angiography. The primary goal is to provide hand surgeons with an organized approach to interpreting arteriography of the upper extremity.

ARTERIAL ANATOMY AND PATHOPHYSIOLOGY
Aortic Arch

The upper extremity vascular system begins at the aortic arch (**Fig. 1**). Although more than 20 aortic arch variants have been described, the most common configuration (approximately 70%–85% of patients) involves 3 main trunks: brachiocephalic (innominate), left common carotid, and left subclavian arteries.[11–13] The second most prevalent formation demonstrates a common origin of the brachiocephalic and left common carotid artery (approximately 5%–15% of patients).[11–13]

Aortic arch disease is often of atherosclerotic origin and involves flow-limiting stenosis or embolic disease to the cerebral circulation and/or upper extremity. A distinction should be made between thromboembolism (thrombus fragment from ruptured atheromatous plaque, sudden onset, and one or a few large emboli) and cholesterol embolization syndrome (microembolic events primarily from cholesterol crystals, less abrupt presentation, constitutional symptoms, and nonspecific inflammatory state).[14] Less commonly, large-vessel arteritis (eg, Takayasu Disease) may be observed, with angiographic findings of long tapered stenoses or occlusions throughout the

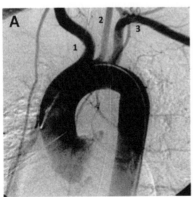 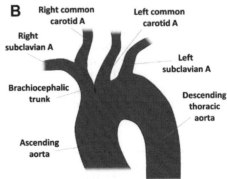

Fig. 1. Aortic arch anatomy. (*A*) Aortic arch arteriogram and (*B*) schematic demonstrating most common arch configuration with 3 main branches: (1) brachiocephalic trunk, (2) left common carotid, and (3) left subclavian arteries. ([*A*] *From* Valji K. Vascular and interventional radiology, 2nd ed. Philadelphia: Elsevier, 2006; with permission.)

thoracoabdominal aorta, its branches, and the pulmonary arteries.[15]

Subclavian Arteries

The right subclavian artery commonly originates from the brachiocephalic artery and the left subclavian artery derives from the aortic arch (**Fig. 2**). In less than 2% of the population, an aberrant right subclavian may branch off the distal aortic arch and course in a retroesophageal position, potentially leading to dysphagia from esophageal compression (dysphagia lusoria).[16] Aberrant subclavian arteries may also be associated with a Kommerell diverticulum, a bulbous enlargement at the proximal subclavian artery that may cause compressive symptoms.[17] Five main branches commonly stem from the subclavian artery: vertebral, internal thoracic (mammary), thyrocervical trunk, costocervical trunk, and dorsal scapular arteries.

Subclavian steal syndrome describes vertebro-basilar symptoms (dizziness, syncope, and stroke) that occur when blood is shunted away from the brain via retrograde flow in the ipsilateral vertebral artery due to stenosis/occlusion of the subclavian artery proximal to the vertebral artery. Symptoms of arm numbness and claudication may also be present. In one study, subclavian stenosis, defined as a pressure difference greater than or equal to 15 mm Hg between arms, was found in almost 2% of the general population.[18] Treatment options include endovascular or open bypass techniques.

Arterial thoracic outlet syndrome (TOS) is the least common (1%–5% of TOS cases) but most concerning form of TOS due to the risk of limb ischemia and loss.[19] Associated bony abnormalities (cervical rib and first rib/clavicle anomalies) may be found in up to two-thirds of patients and symptoms are often masked by chronic neurogenic compression.[20] Other causes include abnormal insertion of the anterior scalene, omohyoid hypertrophy, fibrous bands, and supraclavicular tumors. Imaging studies may reveal aneurysmal disease, stenosis, or occlusion, often at sites of anatomic compression (scalene triangle, costoclavicular space, or subpectoral space).[21] Treatment is directed at outlet decompression with arterial reconstruction as indicated.[19,20,22]

Aneurysmal disease of the subclavian artery is rare (<1% of peripheral arterial aneurysms) and can be classified as intrathoracic versus extrathoracic and true (involving all layers of arterial wall) versus false (pseudoaneurysm).[23] Reported causes include atherosclerosis, trauma (pseudoaneurysm), TOS, infection, and connective tissue disease.[24,25] If left untreated, complications, such as thrombosis, distal embolization, or rupture, may occur. Resection and surgical reconstruction/bypass are often recommended.

Axillary Artery

The axillary artery is a continuation of the subclavian artery after it crosses the lateral aspect of the first rib (**Fig. 3**). Its main branches are the superior thoracic, thoracoacromial trunk, lateral thoracic, subscapular, and anterior/posterior circumflex humeral arteries. Several variations have been described, including a common subscapular and circumflex humeral trunk (<4% in a large cadaver study) and a thoracohumeral trunk giving rise to the lateral thoracic, circumflex humeral, subscapular, and thoracodorsal arteries (<2%).[26]

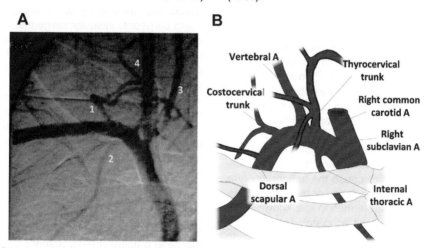

Fig. 2. Subclavian artery anatomy. (*A*) Right subclavian arteriogram and (*B*) schematic demonstrating several main branches: (1) thyrocervical trunk, (2) internal thoracic (mammary), and (3) vertebral arteries. Also note (4) right common carotid artery. ([*A*] *Courtesy of* S.M. Gashti, DO, Medstar Union Memorial Hospital, Baltimore, MD.)

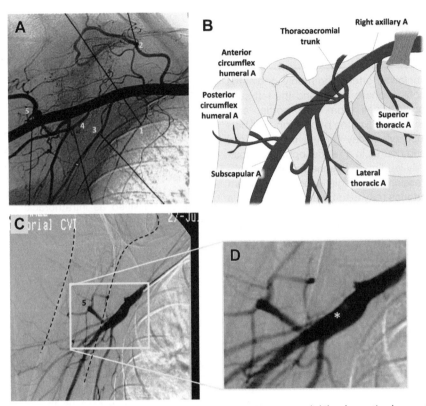

Fig. 3. Axillary artery anatomy. (*A*) Right axillary artery arteriogram and (*B*) schematic demonstrating main branches from proximal to distal: (1) superior thoracic artery, (2) thoracoacromial trunk, (3) lateral thoracic, (4) subscapular, and (5) circumflex humeral arteries. (*C, D*) Right axillary artery arteriogram demonstrating intimal tear (*asterisk*) at origin of circumflex humeral vessels. This injury may be seen in overhead throwing athletes and result in exertional/positional ischemia of the digits. The vessel is injured by traction due to the circumflex humeral vessels leash-like relationship to the neck of the humerus (*dashed black lines*). ([*A*] *From* Valji K. Vascular and interventional radiology, 2nd ed. Philadelphia: Elsevier, 2006; with permission.)

Axillary artery aneurysms are exceedingly rare and are often associated with trauma (penetrating or blunt injury, crutch use, or shoulder dislocation) or chronic repetitive motion. Reports indicate a higher incidence in overhead throwing athletes, who can develop thromboembolic complications from positional compression of the axillary artery and its circumflex branches.[27,28] Intimal damage can be caused by the circumflex humeral arteries acting as a leash around the surgical neck of the humerus. Positional angiography studies have demonstrated transient subluxation of the humeral head during the throwing motion that causes tension at the ostia of vessels from the axillary artery trunk (see **Fig. 3**).[28] Because the axillary artery is a common site for cannulation or bypass grafting, late pseudoaneurysm formation is a known complication that can result in distal ischemia.[29,30] Proximal arterial pathology is generally due to structural compression at the subclavian level; at the axillary level it is more commonly activity related.

Brachial Artery

Although proximal vessel disease is often diagnosed and treated by a variety of specialists (hand surgeons, vascular surgeons, and thoracic outlet specialists), disease at or distal to the brachial artery is more often referred to hand surgeons. Hand surgeons' knowledge of the pathway of these vessels and their anatomic relationship with other structures makes them the best qualified to critically assess angiographic images.

The axillary artery becomes the brachial artery at the inferior margin of teres major and continues along the medial arm in close proximity to the median nerve (**Fig. 4**). Its branches include the deep brachial artery and superior/inferior ulnar collateral arteries. These vessels contribute to an important vascular network at the elbow, including the radial recurrent artery (can flow retrograde to the deep brachial artery), anterior ulnar recurrent artery (to the inferior ulnar collateral artery), and posterior ulnar recurrent (to the superior ulnar

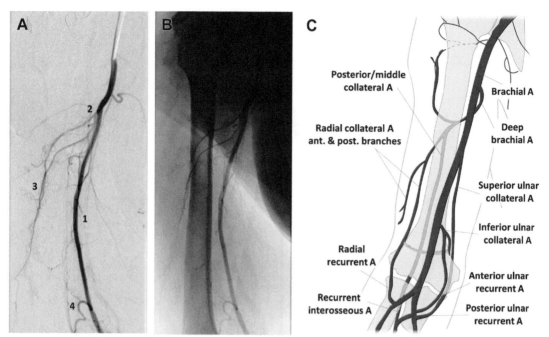

Fig. 4. Brachial artery anatomy. (*A, B*) Right brachial artery arteriograms and (*C*) schematic demonstrating (1) brachial artery, (2) deep brachial artery, (3) radial collateral branches, and (4) ulnar collateral artery. Note position of humerus in unsubtracted image (*B*). Ant., anterior; Post., posterior. ([*A*] *Courtesy of* S.M. Gashti, DO, MedStar Union Memorial Hospital, Baltimore, MD.)

collateral artery). Additionally, the posterior/middle collateral branch of the deep brachial artery can collateralize with the interosseous artery system via a recurrent interosseous artery. These routes of collateral flow enable the distal extremity to be perfused even in the face of brachial artery laceration, thrombosis, or external compression (pink pulseless hand). Angiographic evidence of brachial injury at this level may show increased flow through these peripheral routes.

Distal to the antecubital crease, the brachial artery bifurcates into the radial and ulnar arteries, a common site for lodging of emboli (approximately 70% of cardiac origin).[31]

The redundancy of this arterial arcade permits the harvest of reliable fasciocutaneous flaps. The lateral arm flap is based off the posterior branch of the deep brachial artery (also known as the posterior radial collateral artery) and its pedicle can measure up to 13 cm in length.[32,33] It has been harvested as a versatile free flap, pedicled flap for shoulder defects, reversed flap for elbow defects, and osteocutaneous flap (containing humerus) for segmental forearm bone defects.[34,35] Medially based soft tissue flaps from the superior ulnar collateral artery or distal brachial artery have also been described but are limited by greater variability in vascular supply.[36–38]

Ulnar Artery

The ulnar artery runs along the medial forearm deep to the flexor carpi ulnaris. It can occasionally originate superficially from the axillary or brachial artery but consistently travels with the ulnar nerve at the junction of the proximal and middle thirds of the forearm.[39] Proximally, the ulnar artery gives off anterior and posterior ulnar recurrent branches that can provide retrograde flow to the elbow and upper arm (**Fig. 5**). The common interosseous artery also arises from the proximal ulnar artery and divides into an anterior and posterior branch (relative to the interosseous membrane). The anterior and posterior interosseous arteries have important proximal and distal anastomoses passing through fenestrations in the interosseous membrane that permit the harvest of pedicled flaps for hand, wrist, or elbow reconstruction.[40–42]

Anomalous location, pathway, and origin are much more commonly seen with the radial artery and radial-sided hand than the ulnar artery and ulnar-sided hand. The origin of the common interosseous artery from the ulnar artery, for example, is constant. This is a critical observation when interpreting studies in the antecubital region. Although an appropriately positioned and normal study may be interpreted with ease, 2 abnormal

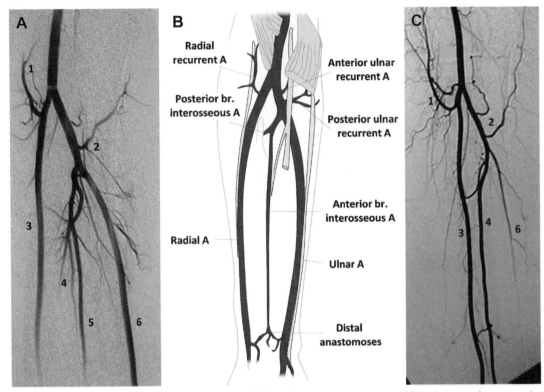

Fig. 5. Antecubital and forearm vascular anatomy. (*A*) Right forearm arteriogram and (*B*) schematic demonstrating (1) radial recurrent, (2) ulnar recurrent, (3) radial, (4) interosseous, (5) persistent median, and (6) ulnar arteries. (*C*) Right forearm arteriogram in a different patient demonstrating distal occlusion of ulnar artery with decreased contrast filling the ulnar artery proximally. Br., branch. ([*A*] *From* Valji K. Vascular and interventional radiology, 2nd ed. Philadelphia: Elsevier, 2006; with permission.)

scenarios may make it considerably challenging. First, an occluded radial or ulnar artery may fail to fill at this level, making the relationships difficult to interpret. In this instance, an anterior interosseous artery (often preserved) may give the appearance of being a radial or ulnar artery (see **Fig. 5**C). Second, nonanatomic positioning of the patient on the angiography table may fool an interpreting physician. Patients may often be malpositioned in pronation (or less than full supination) due to careless technique or patient obesity, resulting in the radial and ulnar systems being superimposed. In both of these situations, the interpreting surgeon should take care to locate the constant and often well-preserved ostium of the common interosseous system arising from the ulnar artery.

At the wrist level, the dorsal branch of the ulnar artery originates approximately 2 to 4 cm proximal to the pisiform and divides into a descending branch (that travels under abductor digiti quinti to connect with the deep branch of the ulnar artery) and ascending branch (that supplies the proximal third of forearm).[43] Up to 6 perforators supply the medial forearm skin along the length of the ulnar artery. Proximal perforators are mostly musculocutaneous and distal perforators run in a septocutaneous fashion between flexor carpi ulnaris and flexor digitorum superficialis.[44] Distally based ulnar artery perforator flaps supplied by these vessels have been described for defects around the wrist and hand.[45,46] These branches of the dorsal ulnar artery can be seen prominently in cases of ulnar artery occlusion at the wrist as a means of collateral flow to the hand.

Thrombosis of the ulnar artery occurs most commonly in Guyon canal, a fibro-osseous tunnel formed by the pisiform, hamate, and several carpal ligaments: transverse carpal, volar carpal, and pisohamate. Risk factors for occlusion include male gender over 50 years of age, dominant hand, history of repeated palmar trauma, and Raynaud phenomenon.[47] Pathologic findings may be consistent with repetitive trauma, thus the designation of hypothenar hammer syndrome (**Fig. 6**).[48]

The ulnar artery is most prone to thrombosis at the distal aspect of Guyon canal (where the vessel is no longer protected by palmaris brevis) before

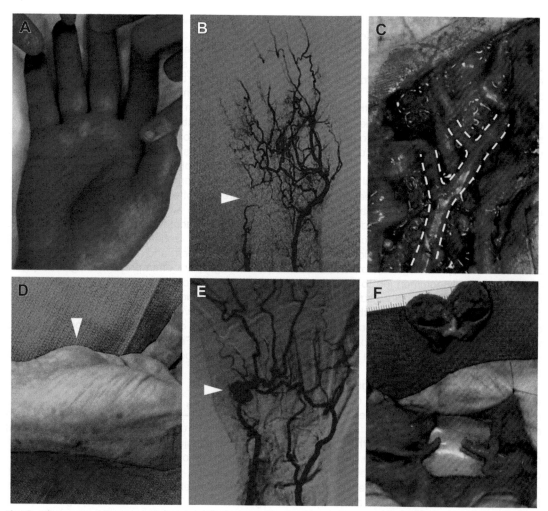

Fig. 6. Ulnar artery disease at the wrist. (*A*) Photograph of painful, discolored fingertips in a 45-year-old dockworker with 1 month of cold intolerance and a prominent ulnar pulse. (*B*) Angiography demonstrated absent filling of the ulnar contribution to the palmar arch and diminished blood flow to the ring and small fingers (*arrowhead* points to occlusion). (*C*) At surgery, thrombosed arterial segments were resected and reconstructed with a trifurcate vein graft (*dashed yellow lines*) from the dorsal hand. (*D*) Photograph of a 2-year history palmar mass (*arrowhead*) in a 61-year-old man with recent blunt trauma to his palm and coolness and pain in his middle, ring, and small fingers. (*E*) Angiography demonstrated an ulnar artery aneurysm (*arrowhead*) with decreased blood flow to the ulnar digits. (*F*) At surgery, the thrombosed aneurysm was resected and the ulnar artery was primarily repaired.

its contribution to the superficial palmar arch. Blunt or penetrating trauma can also result in aneurysm formation, often presenting as a pulsatile mass in the palm. Ulnar-sided digits are often affected and symptoms include pain, cold intolerance, numbness, cyanosis, and ulceration. The proper digital artery to the small finger, which can take off proximal to the hook of the hamate, can sometimes be spared of disease whereas the common digital artery to the 4th web space is usually involved. This may explain why the ring finger often presents with greater soft tissue loss and worse symptoms compared with the small

finger. The ulnar artery in the distal forearm can take on a classic corkscrew appearance just proximal to the arterial occlusion and collaterals are commonly seen at the level of the wrist.

Radial Artery

The radial artery runs deep to the brachioradialis after branching from the brachial artery and continues distally between the brachioradialis and flexor carpi radialis to the wrist. Proximally, it gives off a radial recurrent artery that supplies the elbow region (see **Fig. 5**). Distally, branches from the radial artery communicate with the anterior and posterior interosseous arteries (which also anastomose with the ulnar artery). At the wrist, the radial artery passes in a dorsoradial direction beneath the extensor pollicis brevis and longus tendons and dives between the 2 heads of the first dorsal interosseous muscle. In the palm, the radial artery crosses transversely between the oblique and transverse heads of the adductor pollicis, reaching the deep palmar branch of the ulnar artery to complete the deep palmar arch.

Anatomic variations of the radial artery are not uncommon (up to 30% of patients).[49] These include a high origin off the axillary or brachial artery (**Fig. 7**A), a superficial radial artery that crosses over the extensor pollicis brevis and longus tendons, and the duplication or absence of the radial artery.[50] A high takeoff of the radial artery is extremely common (up to 13.8% in one cadaveric study) and should be suspected when the clinician has difficulty locating the radial artery on angiographic views of the antecubital fossa.[50] When the radial artery origin is abnormal, it is often quite proximal (proximal brachial 65%, axillary artery 23%, midbrachial 8%, and distal brachial 4%).[50] Distal placement of the angiography catheter tip at the brachial artery level can potentially miss a high takeoff radial artery originating proximally.

The radial artery travels through the lateral intermuscular septum of the forearm and provides cutaneous branches (most prevalent distally and proximally) to the overlying skin. The radial forearm fasciocutaneous flap has become a workhorse in reconstructive surgery, in large part because of its reliable vascular anatomy. It has been used as a free flap, anterograde or retrograde pedicled flap, and composite flap containing vascularized bone and tendon.[51,52] Harvest of the radial artery

can lead, however, to hemodynamic consequences that are poorly understood, prompting the development of perforator-based flaps that do not require sacrifice of the radial artery.[53,54]

Thrombosis of the radial artery is often due to iatrogenic trauma (ie, percutaneous arterial catheters). Although the risk of hand ischemia after radial artery catheter insertion is low (<0.1%), temporary occlusion of the radial artery can occur in 20% of cases, potentially resulting in serious ischemic complications in patients lacking a complete palmar arch.[55–57] Radial artery aneurysms are rare and often associated with trauma or infection at the wrist. More commonly, patients present with acute or chronic thrombosis of the radial artery.[58] Ischemic complications, including cold intolerance and ulceration of the radial-sided digits, are often present. Surgical exploration of thromboses often demonstrate a diseased segment throughout the anatomic snuffbox, with the most involved portion underneath its intersection with the overlying extensor pollicis longus tendon (see **Fig. 7**B). This relationship has led some to suspect this as a source of external compression.

Arches of the Hand and Digital Arteries

The radial and ulnar arteries continue into the hand and form 3 major arches that provide a highly variable network of communicating vessels that supply the digits. First, the superficial palmar arch (supplied largely from the ulnar artery) generally gives rise to 3 or 4 common digital arteries (**Fig. 8**). Second, the deep palmar arch (supplied largely from the radial artery) provides 3 to 4 palmar metacarpal arteries. Third, the dorsal arch provides inflow for the dorsal metacarpal artery system. The superficial and deep palmar arches

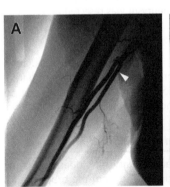 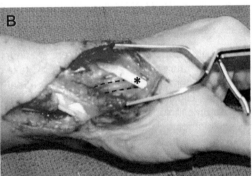

Fig. 7. Radial artery anomaly and occlusion. (*A*) Right upper extremity arteriogram demonstrating high takeoff of the radial artery (*arrowhead*) from the proximal brachial artery. (*B*) Intraoperative photograph demonstrating thrombosis of the radial artery (*dashed black lines*) in the anatomic snuffbox as it exits underneath the obliquely intersecting extensor pollicis longus (*asterisk*).

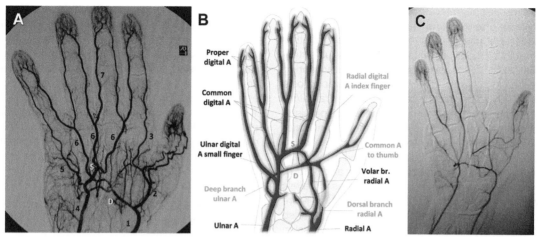

Fig. 8. Hand arterial anatomy. (*A*) Hand arteriogram and (*B*) schematic demonstrating deep palmar arch (D) system: (1) radial artery, (2) common digital artery to thumb, and (3) radial digital artery to index finger, and superficial palmar arch (S) system: (4) ulnar artery, (5) ulnar digital artery to small finger, (6) 3 common digital arteries, and (7) proper digital artery. (*C*) Angiogram demonstrating acute radial artery thrombosis in a patient with an anatomically incomplete superficial palmar arch. Note the division of radial and ulnar artery supply to the digits along the midline of the long finger, with radial vessels originating from the deep arch and ulnar vessels from the anatomically incomplete superficial arch. Br., branch. ([*A*] *From* Valji K. Vascular and interventional radiology, 2nd ed. Philadelphia: Elsevier, 2006; with permission.)

are complete (ie, an anastomosis is found between the vessels constituting it) in more than 80% and 90% of patients, respectively.[59–61] Use of the term, *complete*, has been variable in the hand literature. An arch should be designated as complete if supplied by 2 source vessels. These may include radial artery branches, ulnar artery branches, interosseous vessels, or a persistent median artery. An arch can be *incomplete* if it has lost a second source of arterial inflow due to pathology or thrombosis. A vascular arch may also be *anatomically incomplete* if it has developed without a second proximal inflow source vessel. Incomplete superficial palmar arch development is often observed angiographically. In this situation the ulnar and radial artery systems fail to join along the midline of the long finger ray. An anatomically incomplete arch presents an immediate risk of ischemia when a proximal vessel develops disease/occlusion (see **Fig. 8**C).

The most common type of superficial arch is formed by anastomoses between the superficial volar branch of the radial artery and the ulnar artery. Other variants include an arch formed solely by the ulnar artery, an arch with variable contribution from a persistent median artery, and an arch formed by a branch of the deep palmar arch to the superficial palmar arch.[60] The superficial palmar arch is located distal to the deep palmar arch and often gives rise (from ulnar to radial) to a deep branch that supplies the deep palmar

arch, the ulnar digital artery of the small finger, and 3 common digital arteries.

The most common type of deep arch is formed by an anastomosis between the deep volar branch of the radial artery and the inferior deep branch of the ulnar artery. Additional variants include an arch formed by connections between the deep volar branch of the radial artery and either the superior deep branch of the ulnar artery or both deep branches of the ulnar artery.[60] The deep arch runs deep to the flexor tendons in the palm and is located proximal to the superficial arch. It gives rise (from radial to ulnar) to the digital arteries to the thumb (which are highly variable in morphology and origin), the radial digital artery to the index finger, and branches to the 3 common digital arteries in the second, third, and fourth web spaces.

The dorsal arterial system of the hand is based on branches of the dorsal metacarpal arteries and communicates extensively with the palmar arterial system.[62,63] Studies have shown that the first and second dorsal metacarpal arteries are constant whereas third and fourth dorsal metacarpal arteries are more variable.[64] This vascular network enables the harvest of anterograde or retrograde pedicled vascularized metacarpal bone flaps based on this dorsal arterial system. Additionally, perforators to the dorsal skin also arise from dorsal branches of the radial, ulnar, anterior interosseous, and posterior interosseous arteries.[65]

One clinically relevant arch variant is a persistent median artery (found in 4%–23% of cases in cadaver studies), which may originate from either the ulnar, radial, or anterior interosseous artery (**Fig. 9**).[66–68] This vessel is well developed during embryologic limb development and apoptosis results in its being replaced by the ulnar/radial/interosseous systems. In some cases, it persists, often asymptomatically. It is potentially a major source of perfusion to the hand that often completes the superficial palmar arch with the ulnar artery. A persistent median artery is also known to cause median nerve compression as it travels within the carpal tunnel (see **Fig. 9**B).[67,69] More proximally, a persistent median artery can also be involved in pronator syndrome or compression syndromes of the anterior interosseous nerve.[69]

The arterial system of the digits begins at the common digital arteries that divide into proper digital arteries at the web spaces. Three sets of 4 dorsal branches to the digits have been described: condylar, metaphyseal, dorsal skin, and transverse palmar vessels.[70] Additionally, proximal and middle transverse palmar digital arches

course adjacent to the cruciate ligaments and the distal transverse palmar arch runs just distal to the insertion of the profundus.[70] The complexity of this arterial network has allowed surgeons to reconstruct soft tissue finger defects based on anterograde or retrograde flow island flaps and even perforating branches of the digital artery.[71–73] The arterial supply of the thumb consists largely of radial and ulnar digital branches arising from the common digital artery to the thumb (from radial artery) with anastomoses to the dorsal ulnar and dorsal radial branches.[74]

PRACTICAL ANGIOGRAPHY TIPS
Viewing the Angiogram

Hand surgeons benefit from personal viewing of the angiogram in real time, rather than relying solely on the radiology or vascular surgery interpretation. Reading the angiogram protects hand surgeons from avoiding common errors and allows detailed assessment of the quality of the vascular tree, including the rapidity of vessel filling, collateralization, and retrograde filling. The absence of

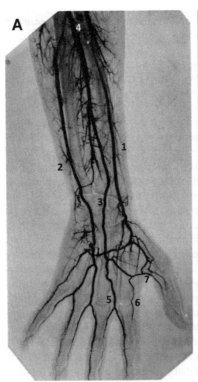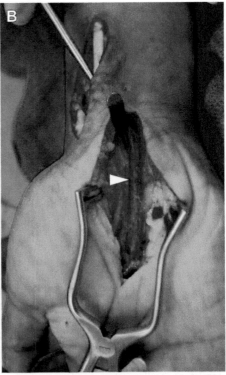

Fig. 9. Persistent median artery. (*A*) Arteriogram of forearm and hand demonstrating (1) radial, (2) ulnar, (3) persistent median, and (4) common interosseous arteries. The persistent median artery appears to supply (5) the common digital artery to the second web space and anastomoses with (6) radial digital artery to index finger and (7) branches to volar thumb. (*B*) Intraoperative photograph demonstrating persistent median artery (*arrowhead*) traveling within carpal tunnel. ([*A*] *From* Janevski BK. Angiography of the upper extremity. The Hague: Martinus Nijhof Publishers, 1982; with permission from Springer Science + Business Media.)

flow on an angiogram does not always equate to a clotted or unusable vessel.

Interpreting the Absence of Flow

The absence of flow on angiogram does not always correlate with a diseased, occluded, or unusable vessel and may instead be reflective of a low-flow phenomenon or elevated back pressure. Occlusion of the ulnar artery at the wrist commonly precludes angiographic visualization of the superficial arch. Surgical exploration in this setting often reveals a patent arch and digital vessels distal to the discrete clot. In general, angiography should be used to discern the location of the occlusion and the quality and caliber of the surrounding vessels, not to determine the extent of diseased vessel.

Care should also be exercised in interpreting the proximal extent of clot burden based on angiographic dye opacification. In a 2- (or greater) vessel system, partial occlusion of 1 conduit may result in preferential flow along the more patent pathway. This may result in reduced contrast flow more proximal than the actual location of the disease (see **Fig. 5**C). For example, in the setting of a radial artery occlusion at the wrist, dye flows more readily through the ulnar artery and contrast dye may only opacify the radial artery as far as the most distal patent small vessel branch (ie, a skin perforator). Although there may be a relatively static column of blood in a patent vessel distal to the branch, this prevents contrast dye from passing distally and gives the incorrect impression that the clot is more extensive than may be discovered on surgical exploration.

Distinguishing the Superficial from the Deep Palmar Arch

Because the superficial arch is often a target for bypass or revascularization procedures, recognizing it on angiogram is of utmost importance. Unfortunately, the superficial arch and deep arch are often confused with each other when angiograms are interpreted (**Fig. 10**). This may complicate a diagnosis and hinder the development of a treatment plan. The deep arch may be readily distinguished by its horizontal trajectory at the level of the metacarpal bases. Additionally, the deep arch is generally located proximal and supplied largely by the radial artery, whereas the superficial arch is distal and supplied largely by the ulnar artery. The superficial arch runs in an

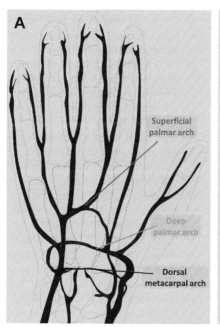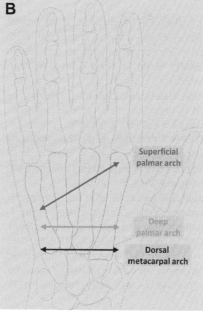

Fig. 10. Distinguishing vascular arches of hand. (*A*) Schematic of hand arteriogram showing 3 tranverse arches of the hand. Metacarpals have been outlined in red. The superficial palmar arch is usually the distal-most arch, originates from the ulnar artery, and runs obliquely across the metaphyseal diaphyses. The deep palmar arch is often proximal to the superficial arch, originates from the radial artery, and runs transversely across the metacarpal bases. The dorsal metacarpal arch may be difficult to visualize but is small in caliber and runs transversely at the level of the carpometacarpal joint. (*B*) Schematic demonstrating the approximate location and orientation of the 3 common hand arches seen on arteriography.

oblique path from proximal-ulnar to distal-radial toward the metacarpal necks and is also much more commonly absent on angiographic evaluation of the diseased vascular tree. Due to the more prevalent complete nature of the deep arch, this is often preserved except in the most severe end-stage disease. The following findings should lead to assuming that the vessel in question is the deep palmar arch: if a single arch is visualized, if it is transverse in trajectory, and/or if it is contiguous with the broad 90° curve of the deep branch of the radial artery.

SUMMARY

Angiography remains an important diagnostic and therapeutic tool that supplements a detailed history and physical examination. Although invasive and requiring the use of contrast dye, it remains the gold standard for imaging of the vascular system of the upper extremity. Numerous variants of the upper limb arterial system have been described and may contribute to surgical pathology. It is paramount to remember that angiography is a dynamic study and should represent a flexible roadmap for surgical reconstruction.

REFERENCES

1. Koman LA, Ruch DS, Aldridge M, et al. Arterial reconstruction in the ischemic hand and wrist: effects on microvascular physiology and health-related quality of life. J Hand Surg Am 1998; 23(5):773–82.
2. Chloros GD, Smerlis NN, Li Z, et al. Noninvasive evaluation of upper-extremity vascular perfusion. J Hand Surg Am 2008;33(4):591–600.
3. Bozlar U, Ogur T, Khaja MS, et al. CT angiography of the upper extremity arterial system: part 2- Clinical applications beyond trauma patients. AJR Am J Roentgenol 2013;201(4):753–63.
4. Bozlar U, Ogur T, Norton PT, et al. CT angiography of the upper extremity arterial system: part 1- Anatomy, technique, and use in trauma patients. AJR Am J Roentgenol 2013;201(4):745–52.
5. Stepansky F, Hecht EM, Rivera R, et al. Dynamic MR angiography of upper extremity vascular disease: pictorial review. Radiographics -2008; 28(1):e28.
6. Higgs ZC, Macafee DA, Braithwaite BD, et al. The Seldinger technique: 50 years on. Lancet 2005; 366(9494):1407–9.
7. Zollikofer CL, Antonucci F, Stuckmann G, et al. Historical overview on the development and characteristics of stents and future outlooks. Cardiovasc Intervent Radiol 1992;15(5):272–8.
8. Murphy TP, Soares GM. The evolution of interventional radiology. Semin Intervent Radiol 2005;22(1):6–9.
9. Wahl S, Lakritz P. Thoracic outlet and upper extremities. In: Bakal CW, Silberzweig JE, Cynamon J, et al, editors. Vascular and interventional radiology: principles and practice. 1st edition. New York: Thieme Medical Publishers, Inc; 2002. p. 7–16.
10. Bucher AM, De Cecco CN, Schoepf UJ, et al. Is contrast medium osmolality a causal factor for contrast-induced nephropathy? Biomed Res Int 2014;2014:931413.
11. Natsis KI, Tsitouridis IA, Didagelos MV, et al. Anatomical variations in the branches of the human aortic arch in 633 angiographies: clinical significance and literature review. Surg Radiol Anat 2009;31(5):319–23.
12. Layton KF, Kallmes DF, Cloft HJ, et al. Bovine aortic arch variant in humans: clarification of a common misnomer. AJNR Am J Neuroradiol 2006;27(7): 1541–2.
13. Ergun E, Simsek B, Kosar PN, et al. Anatomical variations in branching pattern of arcus aorta: 64-slice CTA appearance. Surg Radiol Anat 2013; 35(6):503–9.
14. Kronzon I, Saric M. Cholesterol embolization syndrome. Circulation 2010;122(6):631–41.
15. Gotway MB, Araoz PA, Macedo TA, et al. Imaging findings in Takayasu's arteritis. AJR Am J Roentgenol 2005;184(6):1945–50.
16. Carrizo GJ, Marjani MA. Dysphagia lusoria caused by an aberrant right subclavian artery. Tex Heart Inst J 2004;31(2):168–71.
17. Yang C, Shu C, Li M, et al. Aberrant subclavian artery pathologies and Kommerell's diverticulum: a review and analysis of published endovascular/hybrid treatment options. J Endovasc Ther 2012; 19(3):373–82.
18. Shadman R, Criqui MH, Bundens WP, et al. Subclavian artery stenosis: prevalence, risk factors, and association with cardiovascular diseases. J Am Coll Cardiol 2004;44(3):618–23.
19. Marine L, Valdes F, Mertens R, et al. Arterial thoracic outlet syndrome: a 32-year experience. Ann Vasc Surg 2013;27(8):1007–13.
20. Criado E, Berguer R, Greenfield L. The spectrum of arterial compression at the thoracic outlet. J Vasc Surg 2010;52(2):406–11.
21. Huang JH, Zager EL. Thoracic outlet syndrome. Neurosurgery 2004;55(4):897–902 [discussion: 902–3].
22. Patton GM. Arterial thoracic outlet syndrome. Hand Clin 2004;20(1):107–11, viii.
23. Hobson RW, Israel MR, Lynch TG. Axillosubclavian aneurysms. New York: Grune & Stratton; 1982.
24. Pairolero PC, Walls JT, Payne WS, et al. Subclavian-axillary artery aneurysms. Surgery 1981; 90(4):757–63.

25. Davidovic LB, Markovic DM, Pejkic SD, et al. Sub-clavian artery aneurysms. Asian J Surg 2003;26(1):7–11 [discussion: 12].

26. Saeed M, Rufai AA, Elsayed SE, et al. Variations in the subclavian-axillary arterial system. Saudi Med J 2002;23(2):206–12.

27. Duwayri YM, Emery VB, Driskill MR, et al. Positional compression of the axillary artery causing upper extremity thrombosis and embolism in the elite overhead throwing athlete. J Vasc Surg 2011;53(5):1329–40.

28. Durham JR, Yao JS, Pearce WH, et al. Arterial in-juries in the thoracic outlet syndrome. J Vasc Surg 1995;21(1):57–69.

29. Schachner T, Nagiller J, Zimmer A, et al. Tech-nical problems and complications of axillary ar-tery cannulation. Eur J Cardiothorac Surg 2005;27(4):634–7.

30. Weger N, Klaassen Z, Sturt C, et al. Endovascular treatment of a pseudoaneurysm after an iatrogenic axillary artery injury. Ann Vasc Surg 2010;24(6):826.e9–12.

31. Zimmerman NB. Occlusive vascular disorders of the upper extremity. Hand Clin 1993;9(1):139–50.

32. Sauerbier M, Germann G, Giessler GA, et al. The free lateral arm flap-a reliable option for reconstruc-tion of the forearm and hand. Hand (N Y) 2012;7(2):163–71.

33. Moffett TR, Madison SA, Derr JW Jr, et al. An extended approach for the vascular pedicle of the lateral arm free flap. Plast Reconstr Surg 1992;89(2):259–67.

34. Patel KM, Higgins JP. Posterior elbow wounds: soft tissue coverage options and techniques. Orthop Clin North Am 2013;44(3):409–17, x.

35. Windhofer C, Michlits W, Karlbauer A, et al. Treat-ment of segmental bone and soft-tissue defects of the forearm with the free osteocutaneous lateral arm flap. J Trauma 2011;70(5):1286–90.

36. Matloub HS, Ye Z, Yousif NJ, et al. The medial arm flap. Ann Plast Surg 1992;29(6):517–22.

37. Iwahira Y, Maruyama Y, Hayashi A. The superficial brachial flap. Ann Plast Surg 1996;37(1):48–54.

38. Cil Y, Kocabiotayiotak N, Ozturk S, et al. A new perforator flap from distal medial arm: a cadaveric study. Eplasty 2010;10:e65.

39. Fadel RA, Amonoo-Kuofi HS. The superficial ulnar artery: development and surgical significance. Clin Anat 1996;9(2):128–32.

40. Acharya AM, Bhat AK, Bhaskaranand K. The reverse posterior interosseous artery flap: technical considerations in raising an easier and more reliable flap. J Hand Surg Am 2012;37(3):575–82.

41. Puri V, Mahendru S, Rana R. Posterior interosseous artery flap, fasciosubcutaneous pedicle technique: a study of 25 cases. J Plast Reconstr Aesthet Surg 2007;60(12):1331–7.

42. Coskunfirat OK, Ozkan O. Reversed anterior inter-osseous flap. J Plast Reconstr Aesthet Surg 2006;59(12):1336–41.

43. Vergara-Amador E. Anatomical study of the ulnar dorsal artery and design of a new retrograde ulnar dorsal flap. Plast Reconstr Surg 2008;121(5):1716–24.

44. Mathy JA, Moaveni Z, Tan ST. Vascular anatomy of the ulnar artery perforator flap. Plast Reconstr Surg 2013;131(1):115e–6e.

45. Unal C, Ozdemir J, Hasdemir M. Clinical applica-tion of distal ulnar artery perforator flap in hand trauma. J Reconstr Microsurg 2011;27(9):559–65.

46. Khan MM, Yaseen M, Bariar LM, et al. Clinical study of dorsal ulnar artery flap in hand reconstruc-tion. Indian J Plast Surg 2009;42(1):52–7.

47. Carpentier PH, Biro C, Jiguet M, et al. Prevalence, risk factors, and clinical correlates of ulnar artery occlusion in the general population. J Vasc Surg 2009;50(6):1333–9.

48. Larsen BT, Edwards WD, Jensen MH, et al. Surgical pathology of hypothenar hammer syndrome with new pathogenetic insights: a 25-year institutional experience with clinical and pathologic review of 67 cases. Am J Surg Pathol 2013;37(11):1700–8.

49. Higgins JP, McClinton MA. Vascular insufficiency of the upper extremity. J Hand Surg Am 2010;35(9):1545–53 [quiz: 1553].

50. Rodriguez-Niedenfuhr M, Vazquez T, Nearn L, et al. Variations of the arterial pattern in the upper limb revisited: a morphological and statistical study, with a review of the literature. J Anat 2001;199(Pt 5):547–66.

51. Page R, Chang J. Reconstruction of hand soft-tissue defects: alternatives to the radial forearm fasciocutaneous flap. J Hand Surg Am 2006;31(5):847–56.

52. Martin D, Bakhach J, Casoli V, et al. Reconstruction of the hand with forearm island flaps. Clin Plast Surg 1997;24(1):33–48.

53. Higgins JP. A reassessment of the role of the radial forearm flap in upper extremity reconstruction. J Hand Surg Am 2011;36(7):1237–40.

54. Ho AM, Chang J. Radial artery perforator flap. J Hand Surg Am 2010;35(2):308–11.

55. Scheer B, Perel A, Pfeiffer UJ. Clinical review: com-plications and risk factors of peripheral arterial catheters used for haemodynamic monitoring in anaesthesia and intensive care medicine. Crit Care 2002;6(3):199–204.

56. Valentine RJ, Modrall JG, Clagett GP. Hand ischemia after radial artery cannulation. J Am Coll Surg 2005;201(1):18–22.

57. Chitte SA, Veltri K, Thoma A. Ischemia of the hand secondary to radial artery thrombosis: a report of three cases. Can J Plast Surg 2003;11(3):145–8.

58. Koulaxouzidis G, Kalash Z, Zajonc H, et al. Case of combined thenar and hypothenar hammer syndrome: case report and brief review of the literature. J Reconstr Microsurg 2011;27(6):373–6.

59. Brzezinski M, Luisetti T, London MJ. Radial artery cannulation: a comprehensive review of recent anatomic and physiologic investigations. Anesth Analg 2009;109(6):1763–81.

60. Loukas M, Holdman D, Holdman S. Anatomical variations of the superficial and deep palmar arches. Folia Morphol (Warsz) 2005;64(2):78–83.

61. Gellman H, Botte MJ, Shankwiler J, et al. Arterial patterns of the deep and superficial palmar arches. Clin Orthop Relat Res 2001;(383):41–6.

62. de Rezende MR, Mattar Junior R, Cho AB, et al. Anatomic study of the dorsal arterial system of the hand. Rev Hosp Clin Fac Med Sao Paulo 2004;59(2):71–6.

63. Olave E, Prates JC, Gabrielli C, et al. Perforating branches: important contribution to the formation of the dorsal metacarpal arteries. Scand J Plast Reconstr Surg Hand Surg 1998;32(2):221–7.

64. Dauphin N, Casoli V. The dorsal metacarpal arteries: anatomical study. Feasibility of pedicled metacarpal bone flaps. J Hand Surg Eur Vol 2011;36(9):787–94.

65. Omokawa S, Tanaka Y, Ryu J, et al. Anatomical basis for a vascular pedicled island flap from the dorsal area of the wrist. Scand J Plast Reconstr Surg Hand Surg 2005;39(2):90–4.

66. Singla RK, Kaur N, Dhiraj GS. Prevalence of the persistant median artery. J Clin Diagn Res 2012; 6(9):1454–7.

67. Eid N, Ito Y, Shibata MA, et al. Persistent median artery: cadaveric study and review of the literature. Clin Anat 2011;24(5):627–33.

68. Olave E, Prates JC, Gabrielli C, et al. Median artery and superficial palmar branch of the radial artery in the carpal tunnel. Scand J Plast Reconstr Surg Hand Surg 1997;31(1):13–6.

69. Natsis K, Iordache G, Gigis I, et al. Persistent median artery in the carpal tunnel: anatomy, embryology, clinical significance, and review of the literature. Folia Morphol (Warsz) 2009;68(4):193–200.

70. Strauch B, de Moura W. Arterial system of the fingers. J Hand Surg Am 1990;15(1):148–54.

71. Chen C, Tang P, Zhang X. The dorsal homodigital island flap based on the dorsal branch of the digital artery: a review of 166 cases. Plast Reconstr Surg 2014;133(4):519e–29e.

72. Ozcanli H, Coskunfirat OK, Bektas G, et al. Innervated digital artery perforator flap. J Hand Surg Am 2013;38(2):350–6.

73. Mitsunaga N, Mihara M, Koshima I, et al. Digital artery perforator (DAP) flaps: modifications for fingertip and finger stump reconstruction. J Plast Reconstr Aesthet Surg 2010;63(8):1312–7.

74. Ramirez AR, Gonzalez SM. Arteries of the thumb: description of anatomical variations and review of the literature. Plast Reconstr Surg 2012;129(3):468e–76e.

Index

Note: Page numbers of article titles are in **boldface** type.

Hand Clin 31 (2015) 135–138
http://dx.doi.org/10.1016/S0749-0712(14)00103-6
0749-0712/15/$ – see front matter © 2015 Elsevier Inc. All rights reserved.

hand.theclinics.com

Moving?

Make sure your subscription moves with you!

To notify us of your new address, find your **Clinics Account Number** (located on your mailing label above your name), and contact customer service at:

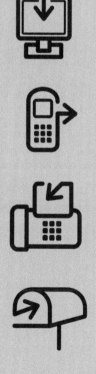

Email: journalscustomerservice-usa@elsevier.com

800-654-2452 (subscribers in the U.S. & Canada)
314-447-8871 (subscribers outside of the U.S. & Canada)

Fax number: 314-447-8029

Elsevier Health Sciences Division
Subscription Customer Service
3251 Riverport Lane
Maryland Heights, MO 63043

*To ensure uninterrupted delivery of your subscription, please notify us at least 4 weeks in advance of move.

Printed and bound by CPI Group (UK) Ltd, Croydon, CR0 4YY

03/10/2024

01040381-0012